TRIUMPH OVER DISEASE

By Fasting
and Natural Diet

TRIUMPH OVER DISEASE

By Fasting
and Natural Diet

Dr. Jack Goldstein (D. P. M.)

ARCO PUBLISHING COMPANY, INC.

219 Park Avenue South, New York, N.Y. 10003

An Arc Book
Published 1978 by Arco Publishing Company, Inc.
219 Park Avenue South, New York, N.Y. 10003

Copyright © 1977 by Jack Goldstein

Library of Congress Cataloging in Publication Data

Goldstein, Jack.
  Triumph over disease—by fasting and natural diet.

Bibliography: p. 237
  1. Ulcerative colitis—Biography. 2. Fasting.
3. Vegetarianism 4. Goldstein, Jack I. Title.

RC862.C6G64   616.3′4   76-44863
ISBN 0-668-04140-4 (Paper Edition)

Printed in the United States of America

Nature understands no jesting. She is always true, always serious, always severe. She is always right and the errors are always those of man. She despises the man incapable of appreciating her, and only to the apt, the pure and the true does she reveal her secrets.

GOETHE

How does one thank those who are responsible for his returning to the human race and to life? It cannot be expressed with words, but my deepest gratitude and thanks are given to:

my dear friend, Carol Leib, who introduced me to the right path;

my dear friends, Dr. and Mrs. Robert Gross, both of whom guided me along that path, picked me up when I was down, helped me when I needed it and showed such an understanding and compassion toward me that there was no other way but to recover;

and my dear wife and soul-mate, Corinne, whose encouragement, optimism, persistence, nagging (Thank God!), devotion and understanding enabled me to take the path. She gave me the strength to go on.

My book is a result of the efforts of these people. It is an experience in living—an enlightenment.

It does not have an ending, because it is a beginning!

Contents

The story you are about to read may seem unreal, exaggerated, and even unbelievable. But whether you like it or not and whether you believe it or not, this is the way it happened. It is truth—every word of it!

Truth is, in fact, stranger than fiction!

Foreword

Dr. Jack Goldstein's book will never be on the required reading list for medical students. Nor will it be read by the vast majority of M.D.'s. Therefore, the patients—and the public—will have to discover it on their own.

And discover it they will! Unless they are content, if they have ulcerative colitis, to submit to unnecessary surgical removal of their entire colon and live with a colostomy bag the rest of their lives. Or, if they have hypertension, kidney disease, arthritis, heart disease or other common chronic diseases, they are content to settle for modern medicine's exclusive answer—hazardous drugs and radical surgery.

"Alternative" is the key word, and alternatives to orthodox medicine are rapidly gaining favor. Decades ago Alcoholics Anonymous proved its superiority over conventional medical therapy. La Leche League, now 21 years old, has established the superiority of experienced mothers over physicians in breast-feeding education. The home birth movement, through its strongest organization, The National Association of Parents and Professionals for Safe Alternatives in Childbirth (NAPSAC), is successfully challenging existing hospital-based obstetrics and hospital-based pediatrics. These, and a variety of other organizations, share with the American Natural

Hygiene Society, of which Dr. Jack Goldstein is past President, a different view of the road to health.

The medical profession is notoriously and historically resistant to new ideas that do not originate with them. I submit as partial evidence of this attitude responses to my nationally syndicated newspaper column, showing the running battle on colitis between this column and physicians:

Dear Dr. Mendelsohn: About two years ago, I began having serious stomach pains with bloody diarrhea. My doctor sent me to the hospital for sigmoid and barium tests, and the diagnosis was colitis. Subsequently, I've been placed on all kinds of medication—Azulfidine, Valium, Prednisone, ACTH shots, Cortenema, Sinequan, Lomotil, and Dyazide. I don't get any better, and a gastroenterologist has even been called in. Doctor, please tell me what this is all about.—M.M., Newark, Ohio

Dear Dr. Mendelsohn: I have been told I have an irritated colon. Even though I have been reassured the problem won't kill me, I am uncomfortable most of the time. I often have severe pains in my right side below the rib cage.

These began about one year ago, approximately one month after I stopped taking tetracycline for acne. I had taken the antibiotic for a year, and during that time my skin cleared beautifully, and my general health improved. Can Tetracycline be responsible for the colon condition?

A pharmacist friend told me that this drug often kills good bacteria that live in the intestinal tract, and loss of this bacteria makes the area vulnerable to infection. If that's true, will my colon return to normal?—Mrs. B.D., Sacramento

Dear Ms. M.M. and Mrs. B.D.: Your letters indicate the problems both doctors and patients face when they treat disease with chemicals. Tetracycline and other antibiotics long have been known to have effects on the normal intestinal tract, and within the last two years, tetracycline has been identified as having negative effects on tissue levels of vitamin C.

As far as drugs used to treat colitis, a distinguished professor of medicine, Dr. Joseph B. Kirsner, who taught me gastroenterology in my student days at the University of Chicago, has written an article in the August 1976 issue of *Drug Therapy* that addresses itself to this problem. Dr. Kirsner cites a Johns Hopkins study showing that drug-associated disease was responsible for 5 per cent of all admissions to that hospital, and 30 per cent of those patients developed a second drug reaction during their hospitalizations. Most of these patients were being treated for gastrointestinal conditions that included ulcers and ulcerative colitis.

Almost all the drugs mentioned in your two letters are implicated in Dr. Kirsner's paper as producing symptoms that often cause the patient's condition to worsen. Also mentioned are Butazolidin Alka, Dilantin, antihypertensives, Indocin, Atromid-S (which causes a tenfold increase in the incidence of gallstones), Elavil, Thorazine, antihistamines and aspirin (responsible for many cases of gastrointestinal bleeding).

I wish Dr. Kirsner's article could find its way into the hands of the many people who are plagued by gastrointestinal problems. He states that the aware physician can help prevent and eliminate many of these drug-induced diseases so that comments such as the following won't have their ironic significance:

Cured yesterday of my disease
I died last night of my physician.—Matthew Prior
(1664–1721)

Dear Dr. Mendelsohn: I am writing this in response to your column on the individual who was not responding to treatment for his colitis and the patient who developed an "irritated colon," possibly secondary to tetracycline.

Antibiotics such as Azulfidine, corticosteroids, Adrenocorticotropin and sedatives, as well as anti-diarrheal and antispasmodic agents, form the basis of the management of patients with ulcerative colitis.

We do not yet know the etiology or pathogenesis of ulcerative colitis or Crohn's disease. Therapy is at best empiric and symptomatic.

Of course, all patients with inflammatory bowel disease do not respond to every type of medical management. This does not imply that physicians necessarily are doing a bad job.

With regard to the patient who developed an "irritated colon" following use of tetracycline, it is true that a number of antibiotics can cause diarrhea and colitis.

The patient in the letter was prescribed tetracycline for a skin condition that I assume was acne, and there was good response. I have confidence that this patient's physician prescribed tetracycline in good faith and felt that its benefits outweighed any possible risk.—Sidney Yassinger, M.D., University of California, Davis

Dear Dr. Yassinger: The letters from patients with ulcerative colitis continue to weigh down my mailman, just as I am sure that patients with this condition continue to fill up your waiting room.

Some patients seem to be helped by the drugs you mention. Others, who are not helped, face the prospect of having most of their gut removed and having a colostomy bag substituted.

The fact that doctors prescribe tetracycline in good faith does not help patients who are damaged by this potent antibiotic. The doctor gets an A for effort but an F for results. God only knows how many drugs physicians are now prescribing, with the best of intentions, that may have lethal results.

Perhaps you and I should call attention to a new book, *Triumph Over Disease by Fasting and Natural Diet* (Arco Publishing Co.), by Dr. Jack Goldstein, a podiatrist.

Dr. Goldstein, a sufferer from ulcerative colitis, was treated by the highest-quality physicians. When medical management was exhausted, the doctors recommended total colectomy.

Instead he turned toward far-reaching changes in both diet and life-style, beginning with a six-week supervised fast, the results of which can be seen on the book's dust jacket—a healthy-looking Dr. Goldstein perched on a bicycle.

Dear Dr. Mendelsohn: I am disturbed at your approach to colitis. I think that you are misleading patients. I particularly was upset with your statement that patients "face the prospect of having most of their gut removed and having a colostomy bag substituted." Using the term "gut" and prefacing it with "most of" is extremely misleading.

The truth of the matter is that the huge majority of patients with inflammatory bowel disease do rather well with medical care. Some, unfortunately, need surgery. I would refer you and your readers to the National Foundation for Ileitis and Colitis for further information.

I also feel that your calling attention to a book by a podiatrist on such a serious disease as inflammatory bowel disease is not quite appropriate. To quote the anecdotal effect of any therapy on one patient as scientific evidence is not the foundation of knowledge upon which modern medicine is based.—David M. Taylor, M.D., Atlanta

Dear Dr. Taylor: If we have learned one basic rule from modern science, as well as from history, it is that truth is not determined by majority vote. Therefore, while patients certainly should not disregard your foundation, which represents the majority viewpoint of physicians who specialize in the field, they also must pay attention to the personal account of those with minority views (even if those views happen to be held by a podiatrist), especially when the method recommended led to recovery after Dr. Jack Goldstein's conventional physicians had insisted that he undergo a total colectomy if he wanted to live.

In a recent letter to me, Emily A. Fine, President of the Greater Atlanta Chapter of the Ileitis and Colitis Foundation, states that some physicians also use the nutritional approach. I hope that the Foundation would give much more prominence to this kind of management which is advocated in Dr. Goldstein's book, *Triumph Over Disease by Fasting and Natural Diet* (Arco Publishing Co.).

I further heard from the National Foundation for Ileitis and Colitis, which advertises itself quite honestly as "a partnership with physicians" (meaning, as in the case of practically every disease foundation, that the patients raise funds directly and through their influence with government to support the researchers).

The "educational" pamphlets that accompanied their letter not only state that dietary factors seem to have little role in the *treatment* of ileitis and colitis, but also completely disregard an important dietary factor, failure to breastfeed, long believed by eminent scientists (Acheson, E.D., Truelove, S.C.: "Early Weaning in Etiology of Ulcerative Colitis," *Medical Digest,* Feb. 1962, p. 116; also Jelliffe and Jelliffe, *Lancet,* Sept. 18, 1976, p. 635) to be important in the *prevention* of this disease. Their letter, accusing me of scare tactics, states: "Ulcerative colitis, like anything else, can vary from being merely annoying to severe. Under no circumstances do the majority of people who suffer from it have to undergo an ileostomy. The percentage is very small. Drug therapy seems to be the best treatment discovered to date, and only as the last possible resort do doctors remove the large intestine. Your column led one to believe that doctors automatically remove intestines after just a trial of drugs, and that is far from the truth. It is only done as a last resort."

Well, I certainly recommend this book for all those thousands of patients facing "the last resort" as well as for the millions who want to avoid ever having to face it. The tens of millions of healthy people will particularly enjoy and profit from Goldstein's rapier-like critique of diets now in vogue (Atkins, Stillman, Solomon, Stare, etc.) and from his excellent section on food additives.

My crystal ball assures me that Jack Goldstein's nutritional approach to disease is someday destined to be accepted by the established medical profession. After all, Alcoholics Anonymous is now incorporated in medical textbooks; La Leche League is today nationally and internationally acclaimed by the very medical organizations which formerly regarded it with suspicion; home childbirth is on the road to achieving respectability; and other groups offering alternatives to conventional medicine are rapidly emerging as public confidence in modern medicine and surgery erodes.

I wish I could have read Jack Goldstein's book as a medical student. I am happy that I know his book now—and that I know him personally. This book—and Dr. Jack Goldstein's concept—deserve the widest possible circulation.

Robert S. Mendelsohn, M.D.

Introduction

It seems the basic tools of the medical profession are the needle, the knife, and the prescription pad. Treatment appears to be, for the most part, symptomatic: injecting of drugs (to do what?), cutting out of parts (end results of disease processes), and the dispensing and prescribing of drugs (almost all drugs are poisons). None of these tools supply the requisites of life. Symptoms are masked; problems are palliated. The patient receives no knowledge or understanding of how to achieve vital health and maintain it. Causes are not removed; and as long as causes remain, then disease, suffering, and agonizing death will continue. The fact that modern medicine has become very effective in the treatment of specific symptoms does not mean that it has become more beneficial for the health of the patient.

Certainly there is a need for qualified surgeons, emergency care physicians, etc. There are times when surgery is necessary as well as the use of lifesaving techniques and drugs. There is also, because of removal or non-functioning of the thyroid, pancreas, or various other glands, the necessity for the substitution of these secretions, the lack of which would result in death.

A doctor is also a teacher; yet how many patients, all of whom have the God-given right to knowledge about their bodies, are ever taught by their doctors the func-

11

tion of their bodies. It seems that the function of one's body is kept secret—a mystery. Why? So many people have told me they've gone to their doctor only to come away with such instructions as, "Get this prescription filled and take the medicine as directed."

People are not taught basic prevention of disease (which, as far as I'm concerned, is the *raison d'etre* of the medical profession), but are taught to expect disease as they get older and to "learn to live with it." But good health is normal and there should be no compromise.

Many of the health problems of today are the result of apathy, lack of interest, lack of knowledge, and a disrespect and misunderstanding of the marvelous innate and built-in wisdom and needs of the human body.

Most people today want instant cure. They don't care how or why they became sick. They just go to their doctor and say, "Doctor, I'm sick. Cure me!" It just cannot work. The body must of necessity eventually break down when it is never-endingly poisoned with drugs. When the doctor tries to improve upon nature, it's the patient who takes the risk.

It is indeed a strange "science" which teaches us that substances (drugs) which make us sick when we are well should be taken when we are sick to make us well.

Nature is slow. It takes years to cultivate ill health because the body can take much abuse, but it also may take years to undo all the damage heaped upon the body by "normal" living. Nature is slow, but nature is sure. One must have patience, knowledge, and understanding.

People have a right to know that there is another approach to health; and this is the purpose of my book. The story can apply to anyone, and anyone can identify and relate to the story. My particular disease is not important; rather it could be almost any other disease, afflicting anyone.

My story depicts the gradual downfall, deterioration, and hopelessness of a person under medical care, with reasons why it happened, and the dramatic recovery when a plan of living was followed (after abandoning the medical gamut) which is in harmony with natural physiologic laws as applied to the human being.

You will learn what is good for your body and what is bad for your body. You will learn a way of living that will enable you and your children to enjoy life—a life of simplicity, free of complication, a life abounding in physical and mental well-being, a life filled with something most people do not seem to enjoy—HEALTH.

Therefore, this book is dedicated to the untold thousands of people who have suffered, are suffering, and may suffer in the future, regardless whether it is ulcerative colitis or another disease, in the hope I can share an experience that could end their suffering, prevent future suffering, and let them enjoy their birthright—vibrant health.

It is my fervent desire that, after you have read this book, those of you who have health will understand how to maintain it; those of you have lost health will understand how to regain it; and those of you who have never had health will have learned how to experience it.

After all, what good is life without health?

PART I

CHAPTER I

Beginning of the End

"I'm dying!"

I was gripped with a sickening fear as I suddenly realized I was dying. What does one do when the doctor pronounces the sentence? What does one say? How does one react?

It was early in 1964. I was 34 years old. I had a lovely wife, two fine children, a good practice as a podiatrist and foot surgeon and was a member of recognized state and national accredited groups of my profession; but I was a damned sick man!

I had run the medical gamut of treatment and by all medical standards there wasn't much hope. I had reached my physiologic limitation as a result of ulcerative colitis, a severe and debilitating disease of the colon or large intestine, marked by severe diarrhea, intestinal spasm, bleeding, dehydration, weakness, weight loss, and a host of other symptoms. It is one of the chronic digestive diseases which, according to the National Center for Health Statistics, are the number one cause of hospitalization and rank second as the cause of disability due to illness. The cost of these ailments is estimated at $10 billion annually, making them the leading cause of economic loss from chronic human illness. About 100,000 new cases are diagnosed each year. Ulcerative colitis is a precancerous state, and it was at this point the doctor granted me two choices—namely, that if nothing was done I would die, or a drastic operation could be tried, a total colectomy (complete removal of the five or six feet of large intestine and rectum), with a bag being attached to the abdomen for the collection and elimination of waste matter (ileostomy), which would have made me a permanent physiologic cripple, and of course could not guarantee my survival. So how does one react when there isn't much hope? I reacted with a calmness, with a feeling bordering on apathy. I almost didn't care. I thought perhaps it was for the better because soon it would be all over. Soon it would end. No more suffering. Eternal peace. But I didn't realize that I was destined to make a decision that was to change the course of my entire life, the lives of my wife and children, and the lives of thousands of people with whom I would cross paths. I was going to hang on to precious life. I was going to defy all the doctors. I was not aware of it at the time, but I was, in a sense, going to be reborn. I had a mission in life!

We have to go back to 1958. I was 28 years old, separated from the army for four years after serving in Korea during the Korean war, had been in private practice only three and one-half years and was trying to make a new start with my wife of two years. It was at this time that it all began—an occurrence which was to become a nightmare and make my life a living hell for the next six years.

My wife, Corinne, and I were relaxing one evening after supper, when suddenly and without warning came a feeling of pressure and discomfort in my lower abdomen, accompanied by strong urge to have a B.M. (bowel movement; the letters "B.M." will be used throughout this story). It happened so fast, there was no time to reach the lavatory and I found myself sitting in a small pool of blood, the sight of which worried and frightened me.

After the initial shock wore off, I decided to do nothing for the present. After all, I didn't seem to have any other particular health problems; my diet was the normal run-of-the-mill American type that lacks nutrition (doesn't everyone enjoy a package of cookies and a quart of milk as a meal, with a candy bar or two for dessert?); and of course I was a worrier, a pessimist, and a perfectionist with an emotional inability to cope with stressful situations—but then don't we all have these "normal" hangups? Normal? I wonder now, as I'm writing this and looking back.

Anyway, I waited three weeks before I worked up enough nerve to see a doctor. During that time, diarrhea developed, accompanied by bleeding and intestinal spasm. This frightened me enough to seek out a doctor who came highly recommended (his real name will not be used for personal reasons, as will not the other doctors who "cared" for me, with the exception of the doctor who finally led me out of the darkness, Dr. Robert Gross).

The initial examination consisted of the usual history taking, blood and urine tests, and physical examination. These things being concluded, I was ushered into a room and told to "hop up" on the table, drop my trousers, and bend over. Dr. Leopold informed me he was going to insert a stainless steel tube up my rectum to visually examine part of the colon (large intestine). I took one look at that instrument, which looked to me like a short stainless steel broomhandle, and asked how he was going to get that thing into me. He said, "Just relax and bear down." But I had built up such a fear and anticipation that it was impossible to relax, and when that cold steel tube (why are doctors' instruments always cold?) touched my sensitive parts and I tightened up every muscle in my body, I knew there was no way he was going to pass that tube into me. He pushed and I sweated. The more he pushed, the more I tightened until finally he gave up and referred me to Dr. Price, an expert in conducting this type of examination. Did he get that instrument into me? You can bet on it! It was probably one of the most enervating experiences I had had to date, and it was to be the first of dozens of this kind of examination over the next six years. However, Dr. Price taught me how to relax during this procedure, which is called a proctosigmoidoscopy, and soon I became an old pro at it, which was to make it easier on me in the years to come.

The diagnosis had been made—ulcerative colitis. A horrible name for a horrible disease. In fact, one of the most debilitating afflictions of man.

Treatment began. If only I knew then what I know now, the agony of the next six years could have been prevented—the agony of a physical, emotional, and spiritual deterioration. Part of the treatment was to find a cause, so blood samples were drawn, urine samples were taken, and I was given a dozen or so small boxes in which to deposit stool samples each week for analysis. Everyone was looking for a germ of some type which was assumed to be causing the disease. None were found, for rarely, if ever, will they be isolated at the beginning of disease because contrary to popular belief—and this may stun you a little—germs are not generally a primary cause of disease. They are ubiquitous and ever present and we cannot rule them out, but their role is secondary. They will grow and thrive in a medium conducive to their propagation, and that medium is an unhealthy body, an enervated body, which mine eventually became. Germs generally won't grow in a vitally healthy body, a body properly nourished and having the highest degree of resistance and immunity, a body that is functioning as it should. After all, what is health? It is merely a state where the body's 25 or 30 quadrillion cells (give or take a few) are all doing their job. I'll go into this later.

Much of the treatment was based on the destruction of germs whether they were present or not. Another aspect of treatment is the assumption that those with ulcerative colitis are supposed to have varying degrees of emotional problems. This is far from always being true. In fact, it is a sick body that usually causes depression and emotional problems as a secondary manifestation.

At this point I was started on drugs, and for the next six years I was to take some forty different types, sometimes gulping down combinations of half a dozen varieties, which when mixed together in my bloodstream caused reactions and crises that made the ulcerative colitis look like child's play. The drugs first prescribed were Azulfidine, for some type of effect on the intestinal tissues; Theragran, a multiple vitamin to replace those lost from diarrhea and the body's inability to absorb the nutrients from food; Pro-Banthine, to dry up secretions such as the fluidity from diarrhea; Trasentine, to relax spasm in the intestinal musculature; Metamucil, to absorb water from the intestines and create a form of soft bulk; and Erythromycin, an antibiotic for an infection that hadn't yet occurred.

Diet was of course regimented. A low-residue type was instituted that avoids roughage, which irritates the large intestine. No raw fruits, vegetables, or nuts. Instead, I used mostly cooked, canned, and pureed foods along with certain meats. This is what I call a diet of foodless foods. Later on you will learn why this type of diet cannot maintain health, much less help recover health. You will also come to understand why drugs do not cause one to get well and that if one recovers health while taking medication, he usually gets well in spite of, not because of, the medicines.

After a number of months my condition grew steadily worse, not so much bleeding now but more diarrhea, intestinal spasm and pain, dehydration, and some weight loss. It was at this point Dr. Leopold decided to hospitalize me. I was there for two weeks, during which time I was given the low-residue and high-protein diet. There were some new drugs administered: Robanul, to hopefully reduce fluid content of B.M.s; Lomotil, to reduce intestinal motility; Sulfathalidine, for further extermination of the non-existent germs; Belladenal, to sort of calm everything down; penicillin, for what was called infection; and Amphojel, to combat the stomach upset and indigestion caused by the other drugs. I was also started on one of the most dangerous of all drugs—prednisone (part of the cortisone family). This is a great masker and suppressor of symptoms while the disease, almost unknown to the patient, worsens. (I'll discuss in more detail later, as I take more and more of these steroid drugs, why they are so dangerous to life.) But what did me the most good was the bed rest.

This was my first experience in being hospitalized and it left a rather bad impression on me after the following occurrence. My hospital roommate was operated on for gallstones. He was quite seriously ill due to cirrhosis of the liver, and the surgery was quite involved. Soon his drain was pulled out, but it was too soon, so he drained internally until he was taken back to the operating room for more surgery. He returned to the room unconscious and with an intravenous feeding tube attached to his arm while a nurse adjusted the flow from the bottle to what was supposed to be the proper drip. But it was much too fast for safety so I rang for the nurse, since he was sedated. When she didn't show, I got out of bed and adjusted it for him. When the bottle was empty, a new one was attached and a new needle inserted into his vein. But it was, by mistake, inserted into his arm muscle. I noticed, as time went by, his arm was almost as big as a football. I rang for the nurse. She didn't come. So I got out of bed, pulled the needle out, applied a tourniquet and inserted the needle into the vein where it belonged. No one ever knew.

While I was hospitalized, I underwent the usual blood and urine tests, stool analyses, and proctosigmoidoscope exams. But now I was to undergo another diagnostic procedure known in the trade as the upper and lower GI (gastro-intestinal) series. This test is done on two separate days. One day is devoted to the upper, where a glass or two of barium meal is swallowed while standing behind a fluoroscope screen as the radiologist watches the substance passing through the upper digestive system, outlining the stomach and upper intestines and showing any discrepancies in the anatomy. No abnormalities appeared during this phase of the examination. The next day I was given the second half of the series called the lower GI or barium enema. This is preceded, as was the upper GI, by taking castor oil and taking an enema the night before. Do you have any idea what happens when, in suffering from intestinal spasm and diarrhea, you swallow castor oil and take an enema? Let's for the sake of brevity, call it an intestinal explosion. The lower GI phase now takes place, which is the infusion of barium by enema, enough to fill all six feet of the large intestine. I was instructed to "hold it all in" while being turned in various positions for fluoroscopy and x-ray studies. If I were to make a short list of the most difficult things I have had to cope with in life, trying to hold in that barium while the diseased intestine was going into spasmodic contraction to force it out would rank high on that list. The physical, mental, and emotional battle that went on during this examination left me totally weakened and exhausted for two days, which further aggravated my condition.

The results of the lower GI examination showed conclusively the presence of ulcerative colitis. The colon exhibited the typical stovepipe appearance, the loss of haustrations (saculations), and resembled a narrow, straight tube. Ulcerations of the intestinal lining were apparent, as were a few polyps (small outgrowths that can become cancerous) which were fortunately able to be snipped out through a subsequent sigmoidoscope procedure.

After the two weeks in the hospital, there was some

improvement, but we must remember that when one is young enough and the disease is in its early stages, there is periodic improvement coupled with periodic flare-ups, until eventually there are more flare-ups than improvements and the disease becomes chronic and crippling. This is why colitis or ulcerative colitis is termed a disease of remissions and exacerbations, and medical treatment is symptomatic treatment. The body is poisoned with drugs. Causes are not removed and the body is never left alone, never given the proper environment to heal itself. Remember that healing is not an art but a biological process that takes place from within the body and nothing from the outside will heal. The body, through its innate power, constantly strives at all costs to maintain homeostasis (balance of all body functions in spite of anything that tends to disturb these functions). Therefore, the more interference with bodily function, the quicker is the approach of the chronic debilitating and crippling diseases of man.

Now came a period of apparent improvement. There were ups and downs through the balance of 1958 and into 1959 and 1960, and in my mind I thought soon the disease would abate. How wrong I was! It was a pseudo improvement—the calm before the storm.

I was seeing Dr. Leopold regularly every few weeks. Minor dietary changes were made at intervals, but I was still in the realm of "baby food." The doses of the many drugs were adjusted from time to time—sometimes lowered, sometimes increased—but I continued to take them to maintain a constant level of these drugs in my blood.

There was, so far, a modicum of normalcy in my

family, professional, and social life. The disease had not created that debility as yet. I still exercised a fairly decent control and probably was "running" anywhere from two to six times per day. Of course, when I had the "urge" it had to be heeded and this began to bother me a little psychologically. I didn't know it at this point, but the disease was to become a veritable curse.

I recall an incident one night in the winter of 1960. I awoke suddenly. A wave of fear came over me. My heart was skipping beats and pounding erratically. It felt as though it would come through my chest. I became light-headed and found myself gasping for breath. I fought hard to avoid unconsciousness. Could this be the end? Is this the way it feels? There was no pain. It was about 3:00 a.m. and I seemed to remember stories of people I had known who had heart attacks. They always experienced them about 2:00 a.m. or 3:00 a.m. As my fear increased, I decided to call my doctor. I apologized for waking him and told him what was happening. He instructed me to call a cab and get right over to the hospital.

"Don't even take time to get dressed," he ordered.

"I'll call the hospital and tell them you're on your way and they'll have everything ready, so don't worry," he added.

"Don't worry?" I laughed to myself. How does one not worry about something like this?

The cab driver was at the door. I told him I'd be right out. I said goodbye to my wife. She couldn't go with me since things had happened so fast and there was no way to have someone stay with our infant son. Corinne was calm. She had an intuition (and her intuitions turned out to be right over the years) that I was not having a heart attack, and that, at least, made it a little easier for me as I walked out the door.

It was a bitter cold night and snow was falling. A hell of a night to go out in pajamas and bathrobe, I thought, as the cab started up. We were speeding, but time dragged and it seemed we would never get to the hospital. Once there, I was led to a reception area where after some fifteen minutes wait (this seems typical in emergency situations) I insisted on someone doing something. No sooner said than done. I was ushered into another room resembling a business office where I came face to face, across a desk, with an efficient-looking woman dressed in white. She coldly inquired as to my type of medical insurance. I got the vibrations that a lengthy interview was forthcoming and I wanted no part of it at that particular time, so I asked to be taken to see a doctor. The lady in white stated she had to have certain information and then I would be able to see the doctor, so she proceeded to obtain my address, profession, phone number, mother's maiden name, religion, and answers to a dozen or so more questions. I almost thought she would ask me why I was there. More precious minutes ticked away and finally the two giant swinging doors opened exposing an orderly who guided me into an examining room and onto a table. At last, I thought, the doctor will see me. Sure enough, about fifteen tension-filled minutes later a very young-looking intern strolled in and asked a battery of questions. He proceeded to examine me and decided to give me an EKG (electrocardiogram); but guess what? That's right! There was no EKG unit in the room. So out he went to locate one. More nervous minutes passed until he returned with the apparatus. He proceeded to put the jelly on the various parts of my body where the electrodes would be hooked up. After connecting me, he was ready to begin. The machine was plugged in, the switch was thrown, but nothing happened. The intern jiggled the switch and made a few adjustments, but still nothing happened. He went to get help while I became more upset with the entire idea. Finally he returned with a young female intern and between the two of them the EKG unit was finally activated, but they could not get the machine to record on the graph. They played with it for a number of minutes—the blind leading the blind—until finally I could not contain myself any longer and got up and showed them how to work it, then I put myself back on the table while they made the test. The results were negative. No evidence of any heart problem. Everything was normal. But after a careful history was taken, it was determined that the entire episode was due to the effects of all the various drugs in my system, each one potentiating the action of another, interfering with normal body function.

This incident reminded me of the story of the man who, when he regained consciousness in his hospital bed, asked the doctor standing over him what had happened. The doctor told him that all of his tiny time pills went off at once.

The point of this whole experience is the frightening prospect that if I, in fact, was having a heart attack, I could have easily died while running the gamut of hospital-medical red tape and laxity most likely due to "routineness." I'm sure this is not always the case, but I wonder how many people have died "waiting"?

My drug doses were of course reduced and altered on subsequent visits to my doctor, but I was ordered to continue taking drugs. Soon I began to experience some nausea and severe general itching as reactions to these drugs. I was then ordered to take two more drugs. One was Dramamine, which was used for nausea, and the other was Periactin, which was used for the itching. Neither of these did much good and there were many other signs of actual poisoning making themselves manifest, some of which were drying of the mouth and mucous membranes, headaches, blurred vision, nervousness (for which the doctor prescribed phenobarbital), mental slowness, and fuzzy mind—probably due to the phenobarbital. There were other signs, but these will give you some idea of the dangers of drugs. This is known as iatrogenic disease, doctor-induced disease, from the so-called "cure," which is usually worse than the disease. In fact, I consider it a small miracle that my infant son, born in December 1960, and my other son-to-be, who would be born in December 1963, were completely normal and had no genetic damage as a result of my system being loaded with poisonous drugs, including one of the most dangerous—cortisone.

After a few more months of treatment, my condition worsened to a point where I began losing weight. I dropped eight or ten pounds from my average 170 pounds. This was of course due to increased intensity of diarrhea, thereby causing dehydration and loss of nutrients. There was also a decreased capacity to digest and absorb food. There was chronic, low-grade fever present, accompanied by malaise and weakness. As the drugs were continued, they caused an alteration in the normal intestinal flora (beneficial bacteria that produce vitamins and are an integral part in the digestive process), creating more diarrhea, vitamin and mineral deficiency, bleeding with subsequent anemia, putrefaction of bowel contents, and resultant gas formation, etc. All of the preceding problems contributed to what was to be a form of malnutrition—another problem I didn't need.

A sick body needs rest. A body that does not have the power to carry on proper digestion needs rest. A body that is weak needs rest. Rest was one necessity that was not supplied. My body was too busy working trying to digest food and detoxifying or making harmless the many drugs being poured into it. How could the body possibly heal itself under these circumstances? The factors necessary to maintain and restore health were never supplied. You will become very aware, later on, of the nature of these factors. The sad part was that I was allowed to deteriorate as far as I did with none of my doctors being truly aware of the conditions necessary for health. From here on it becomes a veritable nightmare.

After two and one-half years Dr. Leopold finally gave up. He referred me to Dr. Evans, early in 1961, who was rated as a "big specialist" with a broader knowledge and experience in treating ulcerative colitis. So I began all over again with blood tests and stool samples, which showed a type of anemia (low hemoglobin in my red blood cells), and the upper GI series and barium enema, which showed worsening changes—and which made me sicker afterward.

After all the above tests were completed, Dr. Evans had me come into his office for a proctosigmoidoscope to "see what's going on in there." He was quite concerned with what he saw internally as well as my generally run-down external appearance and decided I needed some additional drugs. So he started me on Donnatal to quiet things down inside; Combex with C, a multivitamin; Betalin-S injections, a B vitamin which was supposed to give me an appetite; Equanil, a tranquilizer; Haldrone, a member of the cortisone family; and calcium carbonate, to combat the indigestion and stomach upset caused by these other drugs. Of course he cut out most of the drugs that had been prescribed by Dr. Leopold.

My diet was now re-arranged. Dr. Evans allowed me the similar mushy foodless foods, but in addition he advised a very high protein consumption. This consisted of much eggs, milk, meat, and whole wheat bread, which are notorious allergens to many people. A weakened digestive system cannot possibly handle this type of food without having it ferment, rot, and further poison the body. So what happens when a person with ulcerative colitis ingests these? Severe reactions occur such as increased intestinal spasm and diarrhea, mucus formation, and much gas from putrefaction of these foods. I was also allowed coffee, which is a stimulant to the intestinal tract, and I needed that like a proverbial hole in the head.

You can see the inconsistency in medical treatment thus far, which continues as time goes on. Harmlessness should be the watchword, but it was the exception rather than the rule. I saw Dr. Evans approximately once a week for the year of 1961. I was 31 years old but felt twice my age and almost looked it. The proctosigmoidoscopy was done twice at each office visit and was becoming a most uncomfortable and enervating procedure now because diarrhea was increasing to about 12 to 15 times a day, the rectal area was becoming extremely sore, and painful hemorrhoids were developing due to the constant spasms from the diarrhea. This meant it was difficult for the doctor to push that scope past the hemorrhoids.

I could feel myself beginning to crack emotionally. There were periods of apathy and deep depressions accompanied by nervousness and irritability, making it most difficult for my wife to cope with me. In fact, the strain was beginning to show in her. She felt so helpless to do anything for me. She could only watch the gradual wasting away of a once happy and healthy human being.

Since the hemorrhoids were becoming quite painful, Dr. Evans decided to use injection therapy to destroy them. This is a treatment, or should I say torture, where a needle is thrust directly into the hemorrhoids to be destroyed while a strong drug is deposited therein. I thought I had experienced pain before in my life, but this was the ultimate thus far. This I thought was the acme of pain—but I was wrong. I didn't know it then, thank God, but there was still worse to come in the near future.

My fever seemed to be more severe at various intervals. It was becoming increasingly difficult for me to maintain my podiatry practice, to maintain a social life, and even a family life. But I remained with Dr. Evans for another few months until early in 1962. He didn't seem concerned I was running an almost constant fever, that there was infection in the colon area, and that I was becoming weaker and more debilitated. He just went on seeing me once or twice per week and "scoping" me twice at each office visit until I became so abused physically that I could no longer tolerate being under his care. When he began using ultraviolet light tubes by inserting them into the rectum and up the colon, I decided enough is enough and quit.

Being without a doctor was somewhat frightening, but then being with one was also frightening. So where do I go from here? Should I take my chances and try living from day to day without medical help? Or should I seek out another doctor, even though I had built up a fear of them, who might be able to come up with some sort of miracle? I really did not know what to do until some friends of ours, who knew how sick I was, recommended my third doctor-to-be. He had the reputation of being the "best," but he was also the straw that broke the camel's back—he was my downfall.

CHAPTER II

Downfall

It took some time for me to make up my mind to see my next doctor, Dr. Kale, because after all, when you get burnt once and then a second time, you become a little leery about the possibility of a third time. However, an appointment was made to see him. That was like going from the frying pan into the fire for the next two years, until the middle of 1964.

So I began all over again with the blood tests and stool samples which gave similar results as the previous tests except these results showed a general worsening. I was feeling very sick the day of the initial examination. There was a fever and colon infection present, which was probably why I was so weak. Being malnourished from inability to properly digest and absorb nutrients from the food was also a contributing factor.

Dr. Kale gave me a rather long and extensive sigmoidoscope examination. It was quite uncomfortable, to say the least, because I was nervous, tense, and the hemorrhoids formed a slight interference to the entry of that cold steel tube.

What does one think about while this tube is pushed deep into the rectum and colon and moved around at different angles for best viewing? I didn't know what others thought, but I'm sure it was similar to mine. I didn't think of pleasant things and I didn't think of unpleasant things. In fact, I had but one thought: "When is he going to take that damn thing out?"

Dr. Kale was quite concerned upon completion of this examination. No, he was more than concerned. He was alarmed. Alarmed that anyone could have allowed me to reach this present stage without having the common sense to have placed me in a hospital. He informed me that not only was I running a high fever but that a massive infection was present in the entire ulcerated large intestine and was spreading. He said, "I want you to go right home and pack a suitcase and get over to the hospital immediately. I'll phone the hospital and inform them to admit you as a medical emergency." The hospital had no openings for admissions, but the medical emergency had priority. It was one of the few times in my sick life I had "status."

Upon admission I was put to bed and antibiotics were administered for the infection, and aspirin for the fever. The body is trying to eliminate something through a fever. It is part of a remedial process and should not be suppressed by aspirin. Many times, suppression of a fever will result in some unhealthy manifestation elsewhere in the body. Also, the ingestion of aspirin has been proven to cause pinpoint bleeding and even ulcers of the lining of the digestive tract. So why was it given to me? Was that logical? I must attribute my increased bleeding, during the first few days in the hospital, to the always dangerous aspirin. I consider myself most fortunate the ulcers in my colon did not perforate into the abdominal cavity and cause my demise.

My food was called a low-residue, high-protein diet,

which is supposed to build the body and yet not leave too much bulk after digestion to irritate the colon. Most of the food was cooked and pureed, leaving it nutritionally wanting, but this is all I could handle. Put a healthy person on a diet of only cooked foods and eventually his health will deteriorate into disease.

I was advised to have double orders at each meal, if it was desired. That meant double steaks, eggs, hamburgers, chops, chicken, and bacon. Also included in this menu were milk, white bread, coffee, cereals, salt, white sugar, etc. For one thing, as mentioned previously, a sick body does not have the ability for normal digestion and becomes weaker from expending energy in trying. Meat is not good for the body, but is much worse for a diseased intestine. Bacon and eggs are too difficult to digest. Milk generates mucus and creates allergic manifestations. White bread, cereals, and white sugar are highly chemicalized foodless foods and are responsible for many diseases. Salt (table salt, as it is known) is a powerful irritant and has no place in the human body. You know what happens when salt is put on a cut; well can you imagine what it does to a person who has ulcerative colitis. Coffee is a diuretic and stimulant which also has no place in the human body, much less a sick one, and coffee elevates the fatty acid level of the blood while it can also trigger a low blood sugar (hypoglycemic) reaction. I'll try to cover the important aspect of diet in another chapter.

A varied regimen of drugs was instituted during the first week in the hospital. Treatment was always a hit and miss affair, going from one drug or modality to the next and always seeking, always hoping, but never finding. I was going to spend five long weeks in the hospital.

Five weeks away from my family and from my practice, which was already suffering. Five weeks filled with hope —but it was false hope.

Megavitamin therapy began along with a battery of potentially dangerous drugs. There was Sulfasuxidine for infection, Crystalline B-12 injections to combat the anemia, Codeine for pain, Librium for tranquilization, Plaquenil (an anti-inflammatory and antiparasitic agent), Sorboquel to inhibit motility in the intestinal tract, and Maalox for the ever-present indigestion and upset stomach due to ingestion of all these drugs and inability to handle the volume of food.

There were ups and downs the first two weeks, but nothing to indicate any general improvement was forthcoming. Diarrhea was increasing to between 12 and 20 times per day, much of it being just intestinal spasm and bleeding. This, coupled with the poisonous effects of the drugs (nausea, indigestion, blurred and double vision, dizziness, headache, dryness of mouth, and rapid heartbeat), sent me into deep depression, fear, anxiety, and other psychological hang-ups. I was becoming old at 32 years of age and had not enjoyed life for the last four years, at a time when I should have been planning for the future. Instead, the outlook was bleak. I could only foresee a futile struggle to exist—my wife having to work to support us, my physical and now psychological debility worsening until I became a complete invalid (if I lived that long), and a deteriorating family life.

It was at this point in my hospitalization that Dr. Kale began the use of steroids—the cortisone family of drugs. I had already taken small doses for a short time, as mentioned earlier. Thus began probably the most dangerous phase of my treatment with these hormones, the reasons becoming evident, as you will soon learn. Massive doses were given to me by injection and within a few days I began to feel better. The intestinal spasms and diarrhea became less frequent. The migrating joint pains, which can be common in advanced ulcerative colitis, subsided. I began to feel "on top of the world," but these were false feelings of euphoria brought about by the action of the hormones. My appetite was stimulated abnormally and I was able to eat unlimited amounts of food, which was harmful to an already weakened digestive system. I began to put on some weight, but it was a dangerous and unhealthy weight, as will be seen. The severe inflammation throughout the intestinal tract subsided, or so it seemed. But what occurred was a blocking of the body's mechanism to relay the normal inflammatory response, thereby giving the impression of improvement when in reality the inflammatory process was still going on, although I was not aware of it. In other words, while I was feeling marvelous and beginning to "live" again, I was actually dying inside. A very deceptive masking of symptoms was taking place. It was this symptom treatment, or masking of symptoms, that formed the basis for all my medical treatment.

After about a week of these injections, they were discontinued and replaced with tablets called prednisolone (similar to the hormone prednisone I took with Dr. Leopold three years before), which I took in very large doses. I was still taking the other previously mentioned drugs with the addition now of Ananase, which is used as an anti-inflammatory and also reduces swellings.

One of the dangers of taking steroids (prednisolone,

etc.) is the delay of wound healing or the opening up of old sores. So you can see the problem I was up against. I was damn lucky the ulcerated colon didn't break down and allow me to hemorrhage to death. With this potential danger, I could not understand the rationale for using this drug.

The final two weeks in the hospital were spent trying to rest, adjusting drug dosages, taking blood tests and lower GI (barium enema) tests, and of course being on the receiving end of the always-cold steel tube (the sigmoidoscope).

It was sometimes difficult to break the monotony of the five weeks in the hospital, but I read and made friends with many patients on my floor, played chess with some, and even took daily wheelchair rides up and down the hall while pushed by one of my new-found friends. To make the ride even more interesting, I took along my remote control switch from my hospital television set and as we passed each room I activated the switch which changed channels in each room. I could hear various patients trying to get their channels back by cussing and by clicking their remote control units as I went up and down the corridor changing channels. No one ever discovered what happened, but I knew the mystery broke their monotony. Kind of a ridiculous thing to do, but I guess I was getting a little "stir" crazy. These corridor rides were frowned upon by the nursing staff, which put a quick end to an otherwise pleasant daily occurrence.

I recall several other incidents that I look back on now as humorous. It seemed that whenever my hospital roommate would be in the lavatory either shaving or "relieving" himself, that was the time I got the "urge."

When I got that urge I had to move fast or it was too late. After all, I was having from 12 to 20 B.M.s a day. There were many times I had to get him out fast with his pants down. Can you visualize me running in and him running out at top speed and making this quick exchange without bumping each other as we passed through the doorway? Anyone watching would have wondered what the hell was going on.

This particular roommate was to have a sigmoidoscope examination performed in a few days and he was petrified and built up a fear bordering almost on hysteria. He knew I had gone through that test dozens of times and he respected me as an expert. He asked me to give him pointers on how to cope with this cold steel tube. After all, I did know the secrets of these rear-end matters. So I proceeded to coach him in the art of proper mental, physical, and hind-end relaxation. This is the secret of it all. So there we would be, the coach and the student going through the training sessions with him carrying out my instructions. What would the neighbors think if they had overheard the conversation? The day came for him to undergo the sigmoidoscope. He was shaking as he was wheeled out of the room, but I reminded him again to follow my instructions. An hour or two later he was brought back to the room. He was all smiles. He approached me, shook my hand, and thanked me. He said if it wasn't for me, he could never have done it. A simple thing, yes, but it made my day.

Then there were times (it occurred twice) my medicine was brought in while the nurse stood by to make sure it was swallowed. I glanced at the pills and said to the nurse, "These aren't mine." She answered, "These are your pills. I prepared them myself. Your doctor ordered them so please take them." I knew what my pills looked like and these were totally unfamiliar, so I refused to take them until she checked with my doctor. The nurse left the room and was back in five minutes with an apology. "Those pills were for the patient in the next room. Here are yours." Do you know what might have happened if I had not known the difference and swallowed them? They could have killed me. I've often thought of that incident over the years, because it is a common occurrence that takes place every day.

There was a rather pathetic incident I experienced before being discharged. There was an 11-year-old boy across the hall who had such an advanced case of ulcerative colitis that he had to be fed intravenously 24 hours a day. He looked so small, so frail, and so frightened. I tried to spend a little time with him each day, but I could see he was growing weaker. He was wasting away to skin and bones and his doctors recommended a total colectomy—a complete cutting out of the large bowel, with a bag provided to collect the waste matter from a permanent opening in the abdomen. This is one of the most drastic types of surgery. I couldn't see how that shell of a boy, who was listed as critical, would survive whether he had the surgery or not. After leaving the hospital, I tried to get him out of my mind and could not. However, I did not keep in touch. I guess, subconsciously, I was afraid for him and for myself: "There, but for the grace of God, go I." My assumption was that he didn't make it. I almost hoped, for his sake, he did not.

At the end of five weeks, Dr. Kale decided to discharge me. He said, "I'm pleased with your progress." I eagerly departed the hospital with several prescriptions for some of the medication I had been taking, one of which was the hormone drug prednisolone which I was to take in rather large doses for an indefinite period of time, with eventual hopes of reducing the dosage until the drug was stopped. This tapering was to avoid some very damaging and dangerous changes that could take place in my body. I was also instructed to call Dr. Kale in about two weeks to resume regular treatments, which were to be at approximately two-week intervals.

For the next month or two there seemed to be some improvement, or more accurately, a slight remission. There was never really improvement. But I went along, taking my medication and hoping that my bouts with diarrhea, which had decreased to about six to ten times a day, would eventually return to normal and also hoping I would feel better generally.

With this seemingly slight improvement these few months, I became somewhat optimistic and elated. But my elation was short lived because soon the diarrhea increased to about 15 times a day; weight loss was apparent and I was becoming dehydrated from the loss of fluid. I was beginning to run a low-grade fever. Some of my drugs were discontinued and replaced by others, such as tincture of opium for diarrhea (which affected my equilibrium and thinking), Sulfaguanidine for some type of effect on the intestine and bacteria, and Chloroquine for who knows what or why—although it has been used in malaria.

The combination of all the medicines was playing havoc with my stomach, the worst effect being indigestion—severe indigestion. Contributing to this was the hormone prednisolone which I had been taking in rather high doses for a number of months. This drug causes an increase in hydrochloric acid in the stomach. So to counteract these effects, another drug called Gelusil was given. Is it any wonder why normal digestion could not take place even if the ability was there?

The symptoms of drug poisoning were beginning to make themselves evident again: dry mouth, nausea, dizziness, blurred and double vision, fluctuations in mood from deep depression to extreme euphoria, blood cell changes, blood pressure deviations, palpitations of the heart, occasional hot flashes, etc. The double vision made it extremely difficult and frustrating for me to do my surgical work, which was, many times, confined to very small areas on the foot.

As the diarrhea increased, there was more weight loss. There was also loss of minerals, particularly calcium, which contributed to muscle cramps. For this I was given calcium gluconate, which helped somewhat. Dehydration was always a problem and I could feel myself getting weaker. I was drinking large amounts of water.

When the dose of prednisolone was gradually lowered, with eventual complete eradication always in mind, there would be exacerbations to such a degree as to necessitate increasing the dose again. I had been taking these hormones for several years, and very subtle changes, dangerous changes, were taking place in my body. Weight gain was one of them. I had dropped down to about 155 pounds, but now I was noticing an increase. I thought perhaps I was on the road to health. That made me quite happy and optimistic. With this weight gain I experienced alteration in heart rhythm and severe muscle spasms and cramps in my arms and particularly my legs. This was beginning to occur with greater regularity and often with such intensity as to cause my legs to contract and double up. I could not straighten them and I could not tolerate the pain. It would happen anytime and anywhere.

The longer one takes these steroids or hormones, the greater is the threat to life and risk of death, under certain conditions. I was becoming a victim of steroid poisoning. The weight gain was an unhealthy gain due to sodium retention, and we know that sodium holds water. There was also a potassium depletion which was responsible for the severe muscle spasms and irregular heart rhythm. For this I was given potassium chloride pills to try to replenish my potassium reserves.

Other signs of this poisoning were moon-face, buffalo hump, and general bloating. The moon-face is a severe rounding and puffiness, which changed my appearance to the degree that many people I knew could not recognize me. The buffalo hump was deposits of water and fat along the back of the neck. This made me look even more distorted, as did the general body puffiness and swelling. Eventually I reached a weight of 190 pounds. My maximum weight had never been over 170 pounds. I dreaded shaving in the morning because I knew I had to face that monster in the mirror.

This situation continued for a number of months. Right along with it was the continual indigestion which many times kept me awake all night. But it was not just the stomach or colon that was involved. It was the entire body that was now sick; the small intestine, the liver, and other general bodily functions were suffering. What is sometimes overlooked is the fact that the body is one unit. One cannot isolate a part and say this is the sick portion. When a part is diseased or ails in some way, the body is sick and suffers as a unit, even though it is always trying to maintain a balance.

The liver gave me quite a problem. There was always much tenderness in that area. After all, this organ was being taxed beyond its call of duty. One of its many functions is to detoxify poisons in the body. I was loaded with poisons and there was a constant level of these drugs in the blood over the six years of medical treatment. I feel damn lucky I didn't develop cirrhosis of the liver just as an alcoholic might. Just to make sure, Dr. Kale sent me to the hospital for liver function and gall bladder tests. That meant more castor oil, enemas, and drugs—an additional burden to an already enervated, depleted body.

After a number of months, Dr. Kale became quite concerned of potentially dangerous changes occurring and decided to gradually, but very gradually, reduce my steroid dosage. When one has been on steroids as long as I had, and at my dose level, it becomes critically important that this reduction in dose be accomplished over a fairly long period of time. Why? So that the possibility of my dying from shock can be prevented. After all, I've come so far, why expire now!

I feel it important to briefly explain the rationale of this most delicate phase of steroid reduction. One of the secretions of the pituitary gland in the brain is ACTH (adrenocorticotropic hormone). This mobilizes cortisone from the adrenal cortex (a gland lying on each kidney) which is important in carbohydrate and protein metabolism and also in inhibiting ACTH, where each acts as a check and balance system. Another important function of the cortisone is in stress or emergency situations, as I mentioned above. The adrenal cortex also secretes sex hormones.

Now, when this steroid is taken into the body from an outside source over a period of time, the adrenal cortex does not have to produce it, so it becomes smaller and we have what is known as adrenal cortex atrophy. Obliteration of this adrenal cortex can result in death. If at this point of atrophy the exogenous source of the steroid is abruptly stopped, then a most critical situation exists. If a stress or emergency situation should arise—surgery is considered a stress situation—then death can occur from the resultant shock and low blood pressure unless the body receives the hormone from an outside source, giving the body what it cannot obtain from the adrenal cortex.

This was not meant to be a treatise on the subject, but just an awakening for you; to make you aware of the tremendous importance of gradual reduction of steroid dosage so that the gland will "come back" and again begin to produce on its own until it can function normally again when the exogenous source is completely stopped. You see, there are thousands of people like myself who have been in this situation and it behooves us to understand what happens to our precious bodies. I'll tie this in, later on, with an incident that happened to me while I had adrenal cortex atrophy.

My daily intake of prednisolone had reached a peak of 40 milligrams—eight five-milligram tablets—which is quite high. The tapering down was something like one-half tablet every five days to a week. It was a very slow process, but my grotesque size and weight were gradually returning to normal. But as the drug dosage was reduced to several tablets a day, the intestinal spasms increased as did the diarrhea.

I was "running" up to twenty times a day. The other drugs I was taking were not doing much good regardless of how the dosages were manipulated. Dr. Kale did not want to increase the steroid dosage, so he added another drug to my collection called Hydeltrasol—a liquid steroid that I was to dilute in water, suck up into a bulb syringe, and administer by rectum. In this way only the colon area was exposed to the steroid, and we would not have to worry too much about systemic effects. Anyway, I couldn't hold it in long enough to do much good or bad. With so much back-end involvement, some of my friends began calling me the "rear admiral." Not much was funny to me at that time, though.

This method did seem to help to a degree, but it was only symptomatic treatment which was not lasting. The double vision from the other drugs was getting worse, making it extremely difficult for me to perform foot surgery and other intricacies of my profession of podiatry. In fact, it was becoming more difficult to participate in the normal activities of day-to-day living. My life now was completely revolving around my problems almost to the exclusion of anything else. Whenever my wife and I would go anywhere, my first objective was to locate the lavatory and stay within close range. I was living in constant fear and under heavy stress because of never knowing when or where or how fast the "urge" would strike. I didn't live from week to week, day to day, hour to hour or even minute to minute. I lived from second to second.

CHAPTER III

The Agony

The months slipped away into late 1962 and early 1963, but I was no better. My weight came down to about 150 pounds. Here I was, 33 years old in February of 1963 and never had I felt so weak and debilitated. The point had been reached now where the diarrhea would go as high as 30 times a day, accompanied by much colon spasm and continual but varying degrees of bleeding—a classic example of ulcerative colitis.

There were days when I could not go in to work. There were days when I was in my office and did not have the strength to stay more than a few hours before I found it necessary to go home and drop into bed. There were also days where I awoke in the morning and could not get out of bed. But some of the most taxing problems occured in my office, in the car, and at public functions. These problems would have driven any weak-willed or average-willed person to the brink of insanity, and when I look back I wonder how close I did come to joining the "club." Yet as pathetic and mind-blowing as were these incidents, they did have an almost morbidly humorous side.

These things didn't just come and go, but were regular

and continual happenings in my life for many months. For example, in my office, I would walk into the treatment room and greet my patient. I would no sooner sit down when the "urge" would strike and I would have to give some excuse for leaving. I'd return, begin to work on the patient and then I'd have to "go" again. So I'd render another excuse and fly out. This would happen with almost every patient. I've always wondered what some of them thought as they saw me dashing about like a wild man. I don't believe many knew just how ill I was. It was this type of episode which caused me the most frustration and depression, since some of the times, when I had to exit speedily from the room, I didn't make it to where I was headed. I'll leave that to your imagination.

I developed a fear and apprehension about driving my car because there were many times when "nature called" and the usual gas station couldn't be found or the spasm and "urge" came on so fast that it all happened right on the spot. I may be the only person in the world who ever had a B.M. while driving a car at 70 miles an hour. I can laugh at it now, but it was sheer hell then.

It was tough enough to have my podiatry practice and professional life suffer, but it was even tougher to watch what was happening to my family and social life. I was short on temper and patience. I was extremely irritable and depressed. There were many arguments and misunderstandings, all ill-founded, with my wife and three-year-old son. I had changed; changed because my physical debility was finally affecting my emotional, mental, and spiritual well-being. But the pathetic part was that I almost didn't care.

I remember one hospital administrator, a friend of

mine, who observed me at staff meetings over the years. He remarked to me one day, "Jack, you look like death warmed over." Needless to say that remark didn't do much good for my psyche. I wonder how many people with whom I came in contact had similar thoughts?

The simple act of going out to a movie or dinner became an ordeal because, first of all, I didn't want to go. When I finally consented, the strategy had to be planned, such as in what area in the theatre or restaurant would I sit where I'd be close to the lavatory. I wasn't anxious to socialize with friends. In fact, I tried to avoid social situations. But when my wife and I did go to the homes of friends, I searched out the location of all lavatories so as to have a place to escape when the need arose.

I was becoming a recluse. This affected my wife, who needed a social outlet and was also pregnant with our second child who would be born in two or three months— December 1963. She was also teaching in public school three times a week. How Corinne coped with all these stresses without an emotional crack-up still amazes me to this day. A most remarkable woman, as you will come to learn.

Over the years, I have come in contact with many very sick people and heard them utter a statement such as, "I wish I was dead." I didn't have much respect for a person who could make a remark like that. Too dramatic, I thought. But then I had never before been in any situation to warrant that kind of thinking. Never had I grasped the full significance of someone wishing for death. Never, that is, until now. The increasing intestinal spasms, diarrhea up to thirty times a day, bleeding, pain, poisonous effects of the drugs on my mind and body, plus a few other incidentals, had put my life at such a low ebb that I finally did contemplate taking my life—suicide. Suicide? It was difficult for me to realize that here I was considering something I had always abhorred.

The thought would creep into my mind at various intervals during the day, but more often on my "bad" days. As I recall, at this time, in the latter half of 1963, there were no "good" days. I tried desperately to rid my mind of these thoughts, to think of pleasantries and to see things in a positive perspective. But for me there were no pleasantries and I had already become a negative person. Only 33 years old, but I had lived a lifetime.

Corinne lived in constant fear and anticipation that each day I went to my office might be the last time she would see me alive. I don't think she realized the justification for these feelings because she never knew my inner thoughts, my deepest and most private thoughts, although I believe she knew I was capable of causing my own demise. But could I? It was this uncertainty that kept her in a constant state of tension and anxiety.

After all, I did have the means. The necessary pills were in a drug cabinet in my office. Being an expert pistol shooter and enjoying the sport, I owned a revolver. There were many days I would sit in my office and weigh in my mind which method would be better. How would it feel with an overdose? How would it feel with a bullet? I found it impossible to use my imagination with either method, though I finally reasoned that the pills might be too slow. Quickly! That was the way I wanted it to be. The decision was made. Now, do I have enough guts to do it? I knew I could not go on in the same manner. I was tired of pain, tired of suffering, tired of vegetating— I was tired of life.

In my spare time at my office, I would sit back and

fondle the gun, hefting its weight and tossing it from hand to hand. Once in a while I would mockingly place it to my head, then quickly pull it away as if it might accidently go off by some quirk of fate. "It would be so quick," I thought. I wondered if there would be much pain. Even so, "It wouldn't last long," I surmised.

The weeks and months rolled by and I was still playing my little game, but I could not bring myself to pull the trigger. Call it fear, cowardice, ethics, or whatever. Perhaps it was my moral and religious background. I knew that other people would suffer for the rest of their lives— my mother and father, my close relatives, my children, and my wife. I couldn't do that to them. There must be another way. Subconsciously, believe it or not, I still had hope. And there was to be another way soon, a miracle, but not just yet. There was still more agony to experience. It was as if I had to fulfill certain requirements before I could "graduate," before I would be permitted to have body and soul reborn.

About this time, along came another complication which I could have done without—hemorrhoids. This almost reinforced my suicidal contemplation, but it kept me too busy to think about it. I had had some small hemorrhoids during the last year or two, but because of increased rectal spasms and diarrhea with much straining, the small ones got worse and many more developed, both internally and externally. This was accompanied by bleeding and intense pain. The pain became intolerable with each B.M. attempted. I couldn't determine if the bleeding was coming from the ulcerated colon, the hemorrhoids, or both.

Dr. Kale tried to be conservative in the management

of this problem since I was still tapering down the steroid doses. I was advised on hot Sitz baths and instructed to use another drug called Anusol-HC, which is a suppository with cortisone, to be inserted several times a day. Talk about pain! I worked up a cold sweat each time I tried to push one of the suppositories past the hemorrhoids. I eventually had to stop this part of the treatment.

Of course, my ulcerative colitis was still under medical care and the many drugs were regularly shifted from one dose to another. But the most enervating experience now was the fact that each time I would see Dr. Kale, he would have to use the sigmoidoscope. This caused so much pain as it was pushed past the hemorrhoids that I had to be all but held down during this procedure, which left me depleted physically and emotionally for a day or two.

I found it very difficult to sit and also stand due to the severity of the hemorrhoids. The pain was almost unbearable. Cushions did not help. There was almost no comfortable position except over on my abdomen, but this position caused pressure on my colon which forced its spasm, making it compulsory for me to rush to the lavatory.

Dr. Kale was unhappy—but not as unhappy as I— with this situation. He referred me to a surgeon who, after much poking around, decided to needle them—inject them with a medication. I recalled having this procedure performed in 1961 by Dr. Evans and I didn't look forward to having it done again. Anyway, Dr. Cuttem, the surgeon, instructed me onto the table. He told me to relax and then, with the accuracy of a marksman, plunged the needle into the hemorrhoids. When I let out a scream he said, "Does that hurt?" How does one answer a stupid question? With watering eyes I said, "You get up here and let me do it to you!"

This injection therapy was not too successful and Dr. Cuttem hesitated to repeat the treatment, probably at the risk of a broken nose. He wouldn't consider surgery at this time due to the severity of the ulcerative colitis, plus the fact of possible danger from the effects of the still present adrenal cortex atrophy from the cortisone (steroid) drugs. This decision relieved my mind somewhat, because I did not relish the idea of a hemorrhoidectomy. I was referred back to Dr. Kale for follow-up care.

The Thanksgiving holiday of 1963 had just passed. I remember it well because, other than my lovely wife, three-year-old son, and soon-to-be-born child, I had very little for which to be thankful. The onset of what can only be classed as exquisite pain made itself manifest in the hemorrhoid area. I mean pain that caused my eyes to tear. It felt as though the entire "grapevine" was on fire. I like to refer to these hemorrhoids as a grapevine, for sentimental reasons.

For the next week or so, I tried various home remedies in addition to hot compresses. Nothing helped. In fact, the problem worsened in spite of any treatment. The pain grew so severe that it became intolerable. This necessitated my calling Dr. Kale for an appointment to see him immediately on an urgency basis. I was ushered into the examining room where I awaited the arrival of Dr. Kale with my fears elevated and my trousers lowered. He took one look at my posterior, gasped, and said alarmingly, "I don't like the way this looks. I want you to see the surgeon." The fact that Dr. Kale wouldn't tell me anything upset me. So I went down the hallway to the office of the surgeon, my old friend, Dr. Cuttem.

After a thorough examination, which I did not enjoy, including the insertion of a well-developed finger plus a smaller steel tube called a proctoscope, which caused extreme discomfort as it was forced past the hemorrhoids, he calmly informed me that three of the hemorrhoids in my grapevine had gangrene. This was very serious and presented a grave danger to my life.

For some reason I thought back to the year and a half I spent with the army medical corps in Korea during the Korean War. We had seen thousands of problems, including gangrene of the fingers and toes, but never had I seen or even heard of gangrene of the hemorrhoids.

My thoughts returned quickly to the present. I really needed something like this, as if I didn't have enough complications. Leave it to me to be unique. After the initial shock of the news wore off, I could finally listen to what the doctor had to say and it was hardly music to my ears. He told me I was going into the hospital immediately. I called my wife from Dr. Cuttem's office, announced the news and waited as she recoiled (she just couldn't believe anything else like this could happen to me), and told her to pack a bag for me and meet me at the hospital. Corinne was due to have our second child almost anytime and I was afraid all this excitement might trigger things. I just could not visualize her being admitted to the hospital with me while our three-year-old son was at home. Luckily, that didn't happen.

I was admitted to the hospital, went to my room accompanied by my wife, put on my pajamas, and got into bed. Corinne then departed for home. Sometime later, the laboratory technician came in and drew some blood. Then an orderly came in with shaving cream and razor and proceeded to shave the essential parts. I assumed he was rather new at this job because his hands were shaking slightly. I nervously asked him to be extra careful because I didn't want the surgery started ahead of schedule by an accidental slip. He nicked me only once, so I considered myself lucky.

My surgeon visited me to discuss the operative procedure. He said that because my ulcerative colitis was so severe only the three gangrenous hemorrhoids would be cut out. He could not take a chance on a total hemorrhoidectomy with more trauma and larger rectal packing, which I would probably blast right out with my almost uncontrollable B.M.s.

(An amazing thing happened, many months later, to all the remaining hemorrhoids, due to the body's own ability to heal itself, as you will see. This occurs only after I have left the usual medical programs.)

Later that evening, the anesthesiologist came to discuss the anesthetic I was to receive the next morning. It was to be a spinal anesthetic, which didn't thrill me too much. I never did relish the idea of those long, fat needles being pushed into my spinal canal. I was also told I would be given a whopping dose of a cortisone drug to prevent any possibility of my going into shock on the operating table. This tidbit of information also didn't thrill me too much.

Finally, everyone was gone from my room. No nurses, no orderlies, no doctors, and no laboratory technicians. Just silence remained. It was a pleasure for a while, until I found there was time to think. Then all sorts of morbid thoughts came to my mind concerning the surgery and spinal anesthesia. After all, for years I've heard people talk about their hemorrhoid operations—all bad. Now, here I am faced with it. How else could I think? Well, before the evening was over I was completely tensed up over this entire idea of surgery. I could feel the intestinal spasms coming, and before I went to sleep I must have made a dozen trips to the lavatory. But finally sleep did come about 11:00 p.m., at which time I was awakened by the nurse to take a sleeping pill. This was one of the things I found difficult to understand, but when I inquired of others, they told me the same story. After falling asleep, these people were eventually awakened for a sleeping pill.

Morning came and I was awakened at about 5:00 a.m. by an orderly holding an enema. I said, "Is that for me?" He nodded approvingly. There's nothing so refreshing as to wake up early in the morning in a half stupor to have an enema poked into you, mildly crushing against exquisitely tender hemorrhoids on the way in. That's got to wake you up! A few other steps in pre-operative preparation were carried out, which took the clock to about 7:00 or 8:00 a.m. About this time, a nurse entered the room with a hypodermic and said to me, "This is to make you relax." She plunged it into the upper and outer quadrant of my well-cared-for and sought-after hind-end. I knew the only thing that could make me relax was to be anywhere but here.

My wife, my mother, and a friend arrived shortly after the injection. I was so nervous that my hands and feet were blanched, but the sight of familiar faces eased some of the tension. It wasn't long after that two orderlies came in with the cart to take me to surgery. They helped me onto the cart, covered me, and began to wheel me out. I waved goodbye to Corinne whose expression was funereal to say the least. I don't know what was in that hypodermic, but I left the room totally unrelaxed and wide awake. In fact, I really did not want to go, but the intense pain from my posterior kept reminding me there was no alternative.

When we arrived at the operating room, my cart was wheeled over to the operating table where the two orderlies aided me onto it. I gazed up at the large spotlights and then scanned the room. I had always been at the surgeon's position when I performed foot surgery and did not give much thought to the patient's perspective—until now. I was very apprehensive. Soon I was given the injection of the cortisone which would lessen my chances of shock. Then I was rolled over on my abdomen, prepped, and draped. I could never lie on my abdomen because the pressure would stimulate bowel action and I would have to dash for the lavatory. I concentrated very intently on not having a B.M. on the operating table and it paid off. But it did remind me of a few incidents when I had scheduled foot surgery. I was already scrubbed, gowned, and gloved and either ready to operate or already operating when I'd feel a wave of intestinal spasm giving me the usual uncontrollable urge. I would, of necessity, break sterility and get the hell out of there to a lavatory. Then I would return, enervated and embarrassed, re-scrub, regown, and glove again, and continue where I left off.

When I returned to reality from this reminiscence, I overheard two nurses, who thought they were talking quietly, discussing my case. One said, "Is this the gangrenous hemorrhoid case?" The other answered, "Yes it is, and they sure are messy." This did not do anything positive for my morale. It seems when patients are in the operating room, unless they are under general anesthetic, they acquire supersensitive hearing and everything is magnified.

While one anesthetist was strapping my right arm to a board prior to hooking me up to an intravenous solution that would go into a vein on the back of my wrist, I tried to take my mind off it by playing meaningless games. I glanced around at the doctors and nurses all masked and gloved and I thought to myself, "Now I know why they wear masks. So they can't be identified. And they probably wear the rubber gloves so they won't leave any fingerprints."

A sharp pain in my right wrist brought me back to reality as the anesthetist was inserting a needle into my vein to begin the intravenous feeding. I was then jolted by another needle jab which went deep into the lower part of my back between the vertebrae and into the spinal canal. This was to anesthetize the lower portion of my body. First of all, it hurt like hell; secondly, I didn't get anesthesia; and thirdly, I had to be poked repeatedly until the needle was in its proper position in the spinal canal. Then I went "dead" from the waist down and could finally relax a bit because there was no longer any pain. My mind wandered briefly for a few moments and I wondered how hemorrhoids were cut out before the advent of anesthesia. But the thought was too horrible for me to imagine at this particular time, so I returned to the business at hand —worrying.

A syringe full of something was now being injected slowly into my intravenous tubing. I asked the doctor what it was. He said it was a drug to allow me to relax and go to sleep. So I figured I'd like to do that. The anesthetist then said, "As I inject this, I want you to count to ten." I began counting, anticipating a well deserved rest, with my head down and my eyes closed. When I got to ten, I lifted my head and said, "Now what?" "You're supposed to be asleep," the doctor blurted, somewhat puzzled. "Well, I'm not," I responded rather nervously. "I'll give you some more of the drug," he said. So he proceeded to inject another dose into my intravenous tubing. As he did so, he instructed me to count backwards from ten. I quickly thought to myself, "Aha, this must be the secret. I should have counted backwards the first time!" I put my head down, closed my eyes and began to count backwards from ten. Ten, nine, eight, seven —it was so comforting to know that any second I would be asleep—six, five, four—any second now—three, two, one. Within a few seconds, I raised my head and said, "So now what?" The anesthetist, very startled, said again, "You're supposed to be asleep!" "Well, I'm not," I repeated. "I'm as wide awake as you." "I can't give you any more drugs. I've given you enough to knock out a horse," stated the anesthetist. I assumed he was speaking figuratively, because I knew he was not pleased. But by the same token, I wasn't exactly elated.

There is no doubt in my mind that this incident was due to the effects of my body being poisoned with the many drugs I had ingested over the past five and one-half years, some drugs potentiating one another, others antagonizing each other, some neutralizing others, and many interacting. Who knows what detrimental changes occur in our bodies. Obviously, among other things, I seemed to have built a type of immunity or resistance. This was dangerous because it meant I would have to have larger doses of drugs, which can be just as hazardous as being allergic to them.

So during the course of the surgery, while Dr. Cuttem did his thing on my lower end, I chatted with the anesthetist at my upper end. All the while, I could hear various cutting and clicking sounds. I didn't particularly like it, but there wasn't much I could do. After what seemed like hours, in reality it was only about 45 minutes, the surgeon said the most endearing words, "All done, Jack." I was rolled on my back, put on a cart, and wheeled to the recovery room where my blood pressure was taken at regular intervals and I waited for sensation to return to the lower half of my body. The nurse told me I would be here an hour or two, depending on how soon I could wiggle my toes. It wasn't 20 or 30 minutes and I could feel my feet and wiggle my toes. I called the nurse and told her I was ready to be taken back to my room. She said, "Oh, not yet. You must be able to wiggle your toes." "Pull back the sheets and take a look," I told her. She looked and I wiggled. "You're not supposed to be able to wiggle this soon," she said in a rather surprised tone of voice. The doctor was informed of this situation and he agreed to send me down to my room. This little episode was, again, probably the result of biochemical changes due to the years of drugging my system.

On the way down to my room, I could feel the pain starting. By the time we reached the room, the pain was so intense that I became unreasonable and ordered my wife and my mother to "get out of the room." I rang for the nurse and told her to give me something to ease the pain. A few minutes later I received some morphine (¼ grain) and some kind words from the nurse, who was very sympathetic. My wife came back into the room and sat beside me. I tried to keep my mind off the discomfort, but after 30 minutes not only did the pain not ease but it increased in intensity. I rang for the nurse while Corinne tried to hold me down. The nurse said she could not give me any additional painkiller because of doctor's orders. Well, in language not fit to print here, I demanded she locate the doctor and have him change those orders because the pain was driving me wild. The nurse returned shortly with the news that the doctor did not want me to have any more drugs. When I asked the reason, she explained it was because of possible danger to me due to all the cortisone I had been taking. The answer satisfied everyone but me because I had the pain; but that's the way it was. So for the next couple of hours I thrashed around in the bed, screamed, and literally beat on the walls with my fists while Corinne cried and was hysterical in her helplessness and fear.

As all things do, this came to pass and I fell asleep from exhaustion. I was spent. This experience, too, was a result of years of drugging. The amazing thing is that after all these years of disease, of poisoning by the drugs, this hellish surgical experience, and a host of other things related to medical treatment, I had not blown my mind. I still had my sanity.

I awoke early in the evening with the bowel spasms present and an uncontrollable urge to have a B.M. I rang for the nurse; but before she could get to me I jumped out of bed in a wild dash for the lavatory. I didn't make it because the sudden drop in blood pressure caused fainting and I hit the floor! I was picked up and carried to the lavatory where, because of fear, I tried to hold myself back. Finally there was no controlling it and in a few seconds the packing was blown out, accompanied by extreme pain. From here on it was all downhill. The worst was over, but the immense enervation added another emotional scar to my psyche, not to mention the harm to my debilitated physical condition.

Discharge from the hospital came on December 9, 1963. I remember the date well because I no sooner hobbled home and into bed for a well-earned recuperative period, when my wife kissed me goodbye and entered the hospital for the birth of our second son. There I was, left to fend for myself and care for our three-year-old son, when I could barely get around. But my main concern was whether or not the new baby would be born with any mental or physical defects as a result of my system being flooded with poisonous drugs over the last five and one-half years. In fact, Corinne and I debated on whether to have a second child for just this reason. We both thank God that he was born normal in every respect; a little noisy, but normal.

A week later, Corinne returned from the hospital with our new son. We slipped back into the routine of things. I went back to my office and tried desperately to put in as much time as possible, which wasn't much. I found no joy in getting up in the morning to face the day. I had no desire or enthusiasm for my work—or anything else for that matter.

The new year had arrived. It was 1964. I wondered what this year had in store and if it would be as bad as last year. What more could happen to me? I wondered!

But the next four or five months brought progressively worse changes in my physical condition. I celebrated a birthday in February—34 years of age, but an old man. It was tough watching others my age enjoying themselves, taking trips and loving life while I vegetated in my small world.

It seemed there were no lulls or quiescent periods during these trying years. There was always something to prevent an even pattern in our lives. It was very difficult for Corinne to teach school, raise the children, take care of the house, and to try to adjust to my problem. It matured the both of us and that was to our benefit since we were soon to make some major decisions that were to affect the rest of our lives. These years bring to mind Frank Ward O'Malley, the famous journalist, who was asked for his definition of life. His answer was classic. He said simply, "Life is just one damned thing after another." How true!

I saw my doctor regularly every week or two for dietary changes, decreases and increases of my drug dosages, and regular sigmoidoscopic examinations. Nothing seemed to help anymore. The spasms and diarrhea were increasing again and there was more bleeding. I was running to the lavatory 20 to 30 times a day. I was already anemic. Now I was becoming dehydrated and losing weight, having dropped a total of 25 pounds. That put me at about 145 pounds. Low back pain was almost constant and annoying, as were the ever-increasing cramping and spasms in my feet and legs. This was preventing me from obtaining proper and much-needed sleep, since it would awaken me several times during the night and I would find my legs contracted right up against my thighs.

Migrating arthritic pains were becoming prevalent. The aching would travel from one joint to another, affecting several joints at one time. Because of all the drugs I was ingesting, it was all but impossible to take painkillers. If any contained aspirin or even if it was just plain aspirin, the pain and damaging effects on my stomach made it prohibitive. If the drug had no aspirin, and I tried many, then the potentiating effects of the other drugs caused many untoward reactions, not the least of which were confused thinking and a state of stupor. So there was not much I could do except "tough it out." These previously mentioned symptoms are common in colitis and particularly advanced ulcerative colitis. C'est la guerre!

It was late spring, 1964, and I seemed to be heading for what I sensed as some horrible ending. Our family life had dwindled. Social life was virtually over. It took all the physical and emotional strength I could muster just to go to my office and try to do some work. There were more unhealthy changes in my personality. We weren't getting along. There were quarrels. The family relationship was straining at the seams, but Corinne had a bountiful supply of inner strength. Although the body can and does take a lot of abuse, it is astounding how much physical, mental, emotional and even spiritual degeneration can occur in an individual as a result of illness.

This disease, which Dr. Kale called one of remissions and exacerbations, was now just one continuous exacerbation. There were no let-ups; just debility. I loyally continued, for a short while, with the treatment plan until I could see it not only had no value, but was complicating my problem.

I shall never forget my last official visit to Dr. Kale's office. It was probably the most dramatic, indeed one of the most profound moments in my life. I waited for the doctor in an examining room. I felt terrible, but I sat there with hope that Dr. Kale would bring me news of some new drug to cure my problem. (I didn't realize it then, but drugs do not cure. They don't get at causes. Healing is a biological process that takes place from within the body, and drugs only interfere with the healing process since the body must direct its energies toward neutralizing and eliminating these poisons.) Soon, Dr. Kale entered the examining room, sat down with all my records in hand, asked me a few questions concerning the course of treatment and then, after several minutes of thumbing through my records and weighing many things in his mind, he paused and looked up at me. He wore a look of impending doom. Having always been perceptive, I sensed vibrations that what he was about to tell me I had subconsciously dreaded for a long time.

"Jack," he said, "I've done all I can for you. There is nothing more." Dr. Kale did consider a course of treatment, the rationale of which I've never figured out, using a drug called nitrogen mustard, a bone marrow depressant. This was used at that time (I don't know if it is now) for leukemia to drastically reduce the white blood cell count. My white blood cell count was dangerously low from the years of drugging and it was for this reason Dr. Kale decided not to try this method. He did not want to lower my white count any further because of the potential hazard that I could succumb to an infection. (White blood cells are needed to fight infection.)

Now came the moment of truth. This was the culmination of six years under medical care. I turned cold and my stomach knotted-up at what Dr. Kale told me. He said I had two choices: The first was to do nothing, and I would die from the disease. The second was a recommendation to undergo a total colectomy, which is a drastic surgical procedure wherein the entire large intestine and rectum are cut out and the end of the small intestine is sewn to an opening in the abdominal wall. The body wastes would then continually empty into a bag attached outside the body. Having this surgery would not guarantee my survival, but one thing was certain and that was the fact I would be a physiologic cripple the rest of my life—however long or short it would be. (According to statistics from the National Foundation for Ileitis and Colitis, about 25 to 35 percent of patients operated upon require subsequent drastic surgery to remove more of the bowel higher up as the disease progresses.) Neither of these choices appealed to me. Choices? It was more of an ultimatum. Like the old saying goes, "You're damned if you do and you're damned if you don't."

It hit me like a ton of bricks. I couldn't utter a word for a minute or so. It was too overwhelming. I did not want to believe this was happening to me, but deep down in me I knew the score. How would Corinne react? Many fleeting, morbid thoughts raced through my mind. I could not make any decision at this point. The shock of this distorted any rational thinking. I wanted only to be at home with my family now. As I was leaving the office, I told Dr. Kale I needed time to think. He told me not to wait too long. Subconsciously, I wouldn't accept this entire plan. I was disenchanted with the medical profession. I went home to tell my wife. She took the news with a calmness befitting a person with a deep inner strength. Corinne has always been a fighter and she was not about to give up at this point. In fact, she was more determined now than ever before to lick this thing. She didn't know how yet, but there had to be some way. It is just because of this determination that I'm here today and in one whole piece.

Corinne revealed to me, years later, that she knew it would take a miracle to help me; and she was hoping and praying for that miracle, which finally began to materialize as the pieces fell into place in the puzzle of my life.

CHAPTER IV

Discovery

For the next couple of months I drifted along from day to day trying to make a decision. I continued to take the many drugs, which at this point did more harm than good. My diet was very restricted; I was allowed only cooked-out mushes and purees (foodless foods); I had not had any fresh, raw fruits and vegetables for the last six years. But because of the nature of the disease, it was all but impossible to tolerate these necessary and vital raw, fresh natural foods. A normal person cannot maintain health on this type of regime, so how can a sick person?

I was becoming more discouraged and depressed with each passing day. There were always situations which arose to frighten me out of making a decision on radical surgery, such as meeting people who had already undergone this type of surgery. The stories they told me were like nightmares. These people weren't living; they were existing. Sure, there were some that seemed to get along, but they were in the minority. Another situation arose in a department store, where I sometimes went to take my mind off myself. It really did not divert my attention because invariably I would get the tremendous urge to "run" to the lavatory and I would have to stop what I was doing and dash wildly to the men's room, which of necessity I had scouted out when I first entered the store. There were times I didn't quite make it and there were times when I did get there and found people waiting ahead of me. It doesn't take much imagination to realize what happened, but it was a depressing experience and one which occurred frequently and at any time, regardless of my location.

It was in one such department store that I met a friend who was a surgeon. I had not seen him in a while and he remarked how ill I looked. I told him the decision I was contemplating and he coolly told me that he performed this type of surgery. I vividly remember his words of advice as he said, "Jack, if you can avoid this type of surgery, do it at all costs." Well, that stuck in my mind as though it was branded there. I bade him goodbye and he wished me good luck and gave me some parting advice. He told me to "hang in there and maybe one day a drug will be discovered to cure this terrible disease." It took me a while to realize that drugs neither cure nor remove cause.

It was during these two months that a friend, Carol Leib, suggested to my wife that I look into a way of life called Natural Hygiene, which had helped her as well as others she had known. I think if it was not for Carol, I wouldn't be here today—or at least not in one piece. Anyway, Carol planted the seeds in Corinne's mind through frequent discussions, unbeknownst to me. Blessed with an uncanny sense of intuition and insight, Corinne knew that what she was learning from Carol was right. It was logical and made sense, and without analyzing it any further at this point, she knew that here was the help we had been seeking. This was the miracle for which she had been hoping and praying. Corinne had only a superficial knowledge of Natural Hygiene, yet it was enough for her to become excited and elated—more than she had been anytime during these past, depressing six years. She could not wait to finally correlate this knowledge and present it to me.

The day came when she decided to tell me. She was full of enthusiasm and hope as, wide-eyed, she related this new-found knowledge to me. There were numerous facets that made up this way of life, but the two items that stuck in my mind were the vegetarian diet and particularly the use of the "fast" (just water) for the elimination and/or prevention of disease, with the eventual involvement of a high degree of health. I sat there in disbelief. Could this be my own wife advising me to do something which goes against medical principles and philosophy? The very principles and philosophy I had studied years to learn? The principles and philosophy in which all medical doctors are trained? I wouldn't hear of it.

As far as I was concerned, this was some sort of quackery, chicanery. I would not even open my mind enough to read any literature on Natural Hygiene. If it was not medical, I did not want any part of it. I was as closed-minded as much of the medical profession when it comes to new ideas that are revolutionary and may deviate from the dogmatic path. We seem to be enclosed in our own sphere where change cannot penetrate and, for the most part, is not welcome. It is too bad, because there is much help for people, based on principles so simple that it is overlooked by some, looked down at by others, while it stuns the minds of still others who are on such high intellectual levels that they cannot accept or even comprehend simplicity. It took me a number of years to realize this. When I did, I promised myself to keep an open mind and evaluate all facets of an idea. This has opened new worlds to me.

Of course, I continued to receive various suggestions from well-meaning people: "Go to the Mayo Clinic," or "Go to the Cleveland Clinic," or "I know a famous doctor in New York." Frankly, I didn't want any more advice. I was tired of it. I had run the medical gamut and just did not have the desire, stamina, or money to run it again. I also did not want to submit to some of the "heroic" methods being used. I don't believe I could have survived it.

Corinne wanted desperately for me to at least read a bit on this natural way of life and perhaps it would open my mind enough to motivate me to investigate further. But she knew I could not and would not be reached by discussing, nagging, or even arguing with me. So she devised a more subtle approach—a brain-washing without conversation! Let there be no doubt that a determined woman is one of the most powerful forces known.

Every night she would write a little note and put it at the supper table alongside my plate of pills and cooked-out mushes. I couldn't help but see it. There were only three words: "See Charles Dworin." But this was the key that could open the door to my enlightenment. Charles was the librarian of the Detroit Chapter of the American Natural Hygiene Society. He sold the books at the monthly chapter meetings and Corinne wanted me to go over to his house, meet this unusual person, and purchase some of the books.

But each night I would take that small note, which rested next to my supper plate, crumple it, and toss it into the wastebasket. This was usually accompanied by a few choice words to my wife, bluntly advising her to put a stop to this nightly note business. She ignored me of course and continued her little game, even to the point where she would verbally remind me at various intervals during the day. She was a tough woman, but I didn't give in.

So the next three or four weeks found me ripping up notes each night at supper, until one night when I was having a horrible bout with pain, diarrhea, bleeding, and weakness. I sat down at the kitchen table to eat the usual fare, which Corinne had set out for me a few minutes before she left the house for a meeting. She had slipped the familiar note under my plate, but left enough corner exposed so that I couldn't miss it. I had no desire to eat because I was just too ill, but I did stare at her note for several minutes. My children had already gone to bed and the house was quiet—too quiet. The kitchen clock sounded louder than ever as it ticked away the minutes. I reluctantly pulled the note from under the plate and fingered it a while as I studied its message.

Thoughts began racing through my mind as I pondered the note. I recalled these last six hellish years and how life seemed to be ebbing away. Nothing had been accomplished. I also sadly recalled that over these past six years, hardly a day passed when I didn't shed tears over this nightmarish existence. Occasionally, Corinne would hear me in another room and would yell out, "Jack, are you alright? It sounds like you're crying." Of course I responded, nonchalantly, that it was just a coughing spell or some other of a dozen excuses so she wouldn't discover the truth. She never knew. It was one of the few times I was able to hide my deep personal feelings from her. As I read the note again, I thought: "Maybe I will call up this Charles Dworin and run over to his house and purchase a few books. My kids are asleep. Corinne is not here, so I won't have to lose face and concede defeat to her. She need never find out. The kids will be alright since I'll only be gone a half hour or so."

I hesitatingly picked up the telephone and dialed the number, secretly hoping he might not be at home. I tensed a bit when he answered, but I explained, very briefly, my situation. Charles insisted I come right over and said he would get a few books together to give me a start.

On the way to his house, I wondered if I was doing the right thing. "After all," I thought, "I'm a doctor. What could possibly be in those books I don't already know?" As I pulled into the driveway, Charles was waiting by the door for me. We shook hands and went into the house. I felt a bit strange as we went down to the basement where the books were stored, because I observed huge jars of various raw nuts standing about. I had never been exposed to a vegetarian before. Was I expecting some strange looking creature? He looked normal to me as I studied him inconspicuously, so I relaxed.

I wanted to get back home as soon as possible because my children were alone. Irwin was three years old and Darryl was about five months old and they both had birthdays this December of 1964, which was about seven months away. But Charles had such an interesting story about his own experience that I stayed much longer than

I had planned. He told me how he had undergone long fasts and became a vegetarian to elevate himself from the depths of illness to the heights of health.

(As of this writing in 1976, Charles is still the librarian of both the American Natural Hygiene Society and its Detroit chapter. He is still a professional house painter and decorator and climbs ladders all day. He and his wife, Kayla, love to travel and they love to dance. Charles still takes periodic fasts and when you consider he is 74 years young, though he appears a young 60, you've got to marvel at that. He has a twinkle in his eyes and a zest for living.)

Anyway, I purchased four little books. These were all written by Dr. H. M. Shelton, one of the founders of the Society and the most prolific author of books about Natural Hygiene. I thanked Charles and bade him goodbye. I was finally enthused about something and couldn't wait to get home and begin reading before Corinne returned.

After seeing the boys were safe, I settled down in a comfortable chair and examined the books. They were: *Fasting Can Save Your Life*, *Superior Nutrition*, *Food Combining Made Easy*, and *The Joys of Getting Well*. I decided to start with the fasting book, which I immediately opened and began reading, defensively I might add. But soon this defensiveness disappeared and the gates of my mind swung open. This book was not only fascinating, it was thought provoking, enlightening, and it made sense. For the first time in six years I was truly motivated. I couldn't put the book down. Hours later, when Corinne returned, I was still reading. I couldn't hide my elation from her. In fact, I wanted to share this knowledge with her. I could see she was pleased.

Tired as she was from her meeting, and late as it was, Corinne selected one of the books and began to read. She, too, could not put the book down. We became obsessed with the idea we must read all the literature possible concerning Natural Hygiene. We purchased booklets, paperbacks, and hardcover volumes from Charles. I read aloud to Corinne when she was busy, she read aloud to me when I was busy, and we both read independently of each other when neither of us was busy—but we read.

It took several months to study all the material we thought pertinent, yet there was still much to read, but we eventually accomplished the task. I began to realize something so simple that it is overlooked, but I feel it has a definite bearing on our general welfare. This "something" is the fact that doctors study disease, they don't study health. Of course, my mind analyzed these books critically from a medical viewpoint and I found the principles of Natural Hygiene physiologically sound. They are in harmony with natural physiologic laws as applied to man. I knew this was the proper way to live. (I knew it then and I know it now—only with more conviction.)

It was late summer 1964 when I made my decision. I had to get involved in this natural way of life. I had the book knowledge and academic background, but now it had to be used, to be put into practice and experienced. Knowledge and experience must go hand-in-hand to form a symbiosis—a partnership. But how does one get involved? Who does one contact?

My friend, Carol Leib, recommended Dr. Robert Gross in Hyde Park, New York, because she knew him and had undergone fasts under his supervision. (There are Hygienic practitioners located around the country, all qualified and experienced, and I have come to know and love every one of them.) So I put together a letter informing Dr. Gross of my case history and expressing a desire to put myself under his care. I wondered how long it would take for him to answer. I was hoping it would be soon, because time was becoming a critical factor. I had dropped another five pounds and was down to 140 pounds, giving me a total loss of 30 pounds.

A week or ten days later, Corinne called me at my office. She was excited because, as I had already deduced, a letter arrived from Dr. Gross. Corinne wanted to open it, but I said no. I wanted to be the first to read it. The day couldn't pass fast enough for me now. The clock seemed to stand still as a punishment to me for watching it so closely. I couldn't wait until my last patient left the office so I could rush home and open that letter.

The drive home seemed to take longer than usual. The traffic seemed heavier and the distance further, but finally I was pulling in the driveway. I left the car and was through the front door of my home in record time. Corinne handed me the letter, anxiously watching as I opened it. I sat down and began to read. What my eyes saw, my mind refused to believe. I re-read the letter. Dr. Gross would not accept me as a patient.

If I had been on the brink of a nervous breakdown, this letter would have nudged me over the edge. I had mixed emotions: disgust, anger, depression, disappointment, and even self-pity. I was stunned; couldn't think rationally. It took a lot of strength to keep from bursting out crying at the realization that my last hopes were gone.

I decided that within the next couple of days I was going to make an appointment with the surgeon and have my "insides" cut out, because I could no longer tolerate this type of existence. However, within these next couple of days I received correspondence from Dr. Gross. He told me to disregard the previous letter and that I should come to Pawling Health Manor if I still wished it, but to be prepared to spend three months away from home. Naturally, no guarantees were made; but he said as long as I was so determined, he was willing to work with me. I was elated! I felt I belonged to the human race again. After all, there was nothing to lose and everything to gain. I could always come back and have the operation if this failed, but I could not, with a clear conscience, undergo the surgery without first trying this last hope. Once the colon and rectum are cut out, they cannot be put back.

(Bob Gross and I developed a very close relationship over the years. It was after this relationship was established that Bob explained the reason for his initial refusal to accept me as a patient. To put it tersely, he thought because of the gravity of my physical condition, that I might die at the Manor. But there were several things in my favor that prompted him to take a chance: I still had youth and I had that all-important drive and determination to recover. But one other important factor played a key role, which I discovered for myself—Dr. Gross' deep compassion for the welfare of a human being.)

I began planning for my three-month exile. Personal and private matters were settled, my wife and I discussed her getting along without me, and a very close friend, Dr. Newton Karp, offered to give up his day off plus one working day to run my office two days a week so I wouldn't lose my practice. Our other friends and relatives assured me they would look after my family while I was away—and they surely did!

During the interval between making arrangements for my departure and the actual departure, I received phone calls from various well-meaning relatives and friends. They said such things as, "You're crazy—don't do it"; "You're making a mistake"; "It's quackery"; etc., etc. There were many other negative bits of advice given. But there were a few people who congratulated me on having enough courage to make a decision to break away from the "herd." Why is it that the biggest critics are usually those who know little or nothing about what they are criticizing?

Advance train reservations were made and I was ready to go. The train was to depart from the Michigan Central Depot about 7:00 p.m. on September 2, 1964. The trip would take about 13 hours, arriving in Poughkeepsie, New York, at 8:00 a.m. the following morning. Poughkeepsie is about 15 miles south of Hyde Park and is the closest stop. It is necessary to take a northbound train back past Hyde Park and into Rhinecliff, which is five or six miles from Pawling Health Manor at the extreme north end of Hyde Park. A taxi is then taken direct to the Manor.

I started saying my goodbyes several days before leaving. I took time to visit Dr. Kale and told him my plans. He said he couldn't see me wasting my time, but he did concede that if I was not going to be put on drugs (which I definitely was not—in fact, this plan of living shuns drugs and other poisons) and I was not going to eat (fasting) for a while, then it shouldn't be harmful. But Dr. Kale would not concede, in the slightest, that I could possibly be helped. I did discover that Dr. Kale told another doctor that I would be back to have the operation.

The dawn of September 2 made its appearance. I was awakened by the sunlight streaming in through the window and dancing off the walls. I was very tired, since I slept poorly. It was the anticipation of what was to come, plus the fact it was my last night at home for at least three months. Running to the lavatory half the night didn't help matters any; neither did the half-dozen trips on awakening—another characteristic and daily occurrence for those with ulcerative colitis.

Finally I got down to the business of packing. I began early because I wanted to be sure I had everything I would need for the next three months, including plenty of stationery, some light reading materials, a chess set, and a small radio with an ear plug. Other than the packing, it was a rather quiet day. I was somewhat nervous, but it was calming just to be with my family these last few hours.

As train time drew closer, I began having second thoughts. I wondered if I was doing the right thing. I wondered if I'd ever come back. It was all so new to me; so anti-establishment. This Natural Hygiene way of life seemed to go contrary to many things I had been taught (brainwashed?) during my life. Did that make it wrong? Everything I had read and analyzed convinced me it was right and I had to realize that, even with truth on my side, it would be difficult to travel upstream against the current of society's one-way flow.

I left my house one hour before train time, accompanied by an entourage consisting of my mother and father, my mother-in-law and father-in-law, and my wife and two sons. A solemn atmosphere prevailed during the drive to the depot, which bore a resemblance to a funeral procession. Everything was running like clockwork. It was too good to be true. That's probably why there was a blowout in one of the front tires when we were halfway to the train station. At least things seemed back to the normal confusion. It must have been a sight for passing motorists to see all of us scurrying out and around the car. Not having learned the art of emotional poise yet, I worked up a nervous sweat and became so tense, for fear of missing my train, that I thought I'd have a B.M. right there on the expressway. This had to be one of the fastest tire changes on record for a family car. We jumped back into the car and off we went, the solemnity now broken by this humorous, yet not-so-humorous, incident.

We arrived about 15 minutes before departure, so all of us walked over to the track where the train was waiting. We engaged in small talk for a while, until the conductor bellowed his, "All aboard." My heart began pounding as I said goodbye to everyone, especially my wife and children. (My mother-in-law revealed to me only recently how frail I looked as I boarded the train and she wondered if I would ever come back. Quite frankly, so did I.)

As the train inched forward, we all began waving frantically and I wanted to get off. My parents and in-laws were crying as the moving train put a little more distance between us. Corinne didn't cry. She didn't, because she was happy for me, relieved for me. Corinne was optmistic and confident and knew in her heart that everything was going to work out. I continued watching through the window until the increasing distance made them all disappear. Then I sat back, unmoving for about ten minutes, and burst out crying. It was a release that finally allowed me to relax.

(Corinne told me, years later, there were many times she cried at home while I was away. This occurred only when her confidence in what I was doing was shaken by someone challenging her on this natural lifestyle. She didn't know enough about it to defend it at this point, so she was easily swayed by well-meaning people, all of whom were misinformed or had no knowledge on which to base their advice. Each time these incidents would occur, it would leave her panicky and somewhat hysterical, thinking I had made a terrible mistake. Yet, deep down, an inner voice gave her strength and faith to overcome these obstacles and she came away from these experiences more imbued with the truth of what I was doing.)

I had taken a roomette on the train, which is a tiny private room with a sink, a pull-down bed, and a single seat. The fascinating thing is when this seat is raised, there's the toilet. This was heaven for me, but I think I spent more time sitting with the seat up. I felt secure being enclosed in this little room, gazing out the window and watching the changing scenes as the train whizzed along. I was enjoying the solitude, the absence of people, and the monotonous clickety-clack of the wheels as they passed over the seams in the track.

I thought about the next three months. I knew I was going to be put on a fast, but I didn't know for how long. I tried to imagine what it would be like to abstain from food, with the exception of water, for a length of time, but I could not visualize it in my mind's eye. I knew, if I survived this undertaking, I would become a vegetarian. I wondered how that would feel, as I reached over for my bag of food.

The fact that I was relaxed and not tense contributed to a desire to eat. Knowing I was to become a vegetarian, I filled this large bag at home with what I called, ironically, the "Last Supper"! There were cold lamb chops, chicken, roast beef, hamburger, breaded veal cutlet, and I don't remember what else. I figured I should eat all this to fortify myself against the ensuing meatless years. Well, I ate and ate and ate some more until I became so ill that for ten minutes I vomited everything I had swallowed. This took all the strength out of me.

I decided to pull down the bed and get to sleep early. Besides, it was dark out now and there wasn't much to see. I put on my pajamas, jumped into bed, turned out the light, and lay there staring out the window. It was a nice feeling watching the multi-colored lights of cities at night blink by. I loved to hear the low sound of the rail-road-crossing bells in the distance gradually becoming louder and louder until we passed them; then they gradually faded away in the distance. I didn't sleep too well because I couldn't clear my mind, which was very active all night.

I watched the dawn break and the sun peek over the hills. I knew this day, September 3, 1964, was to be a special day for me. I dressed and shaved quickly and straightened my roomette. Then I sat back and waited for our arrival. We had been travelling adjacent to the Hudson river for many miles, while the sun darted in and out from between the hills, occasionally sending dazzling reflections bouncing off the river's calm, morning glassiness. There was a tranquility in watching the gentle, ever-changing scenery as the river meandered and cut its way through the lush, green mountainous foothills. All along the banks of the Hudson, people could be seen fishing. Some had built bonfires to chase away the early morning chill. I envisioned myself out there without a care in the world.

A loud knock at the door startled me out of my fantasy as the conductor operatically announced Poughkeepsie. I glanced at my watch. Almost 8:00 a.m. We should be arriving close to the scheduled time, although I can't recall ever being on a train that was on time. This one didn't break any precedent as we came to a stop at the Poughkeepsie station about 8:20 a.m.—20 minutes late, which gave me ten minutes to struggle off the train with my luggage, run into the depot and purchase a ticket back to Rhinecliff and hurry breathlessly back onto the waiting platform with probably only seconds to spare. However, this would not become a problem because, true to form, the train was a half-hour late.

The 25 minute ride back up the Hudson river was uneventful. The same people seemed to be fishing in the same places. Rhinecliff station was announced and when the train stopped I maneuvered my luggage off and hailed a cab. The driver saw how weak I was, so he graciously herded me and the suitcases into his car and off we went six miles downriver again. We passed through Rhinecliff, Rhinebeck, and into the northern end of Hyde Park, where Pawling Health Manor was located.

As we drove onto the grounds, I could appreciate the beauty of this part of the country. The main house was situated on a hill and surrounded by trees of many species. There was a commanding view of the Hudson River with the mountains for a backdrop. This looked like a place one could rest. There were people scattered around, sitting in the sun.

The cab came to a stop in front of the Manor and I stepped out. I took a deep breath. The crisp morning air was clean and sweet. It was actually breathable. I took in another deep breath. This air was so different from the polluted stuff I had become accustomed to back home in the Detroit area.

As I walked up the few short steps to the front door, I wondered what fate had in store for me.

CHAPTER V

My Six Week Fast

Once inside this three-storied mansion, I observed people who were in varying lengths of a fast and people who had already broken their fasts and had been eating. It seems they were all discussing one subject—food. (Later on, I too would succumb to this pastime.) I noticed the furnishings were modest and there was a cleanliness that shone throughout. There was a characteristic aroma which permeated the air. It was from a marvelous vegetable soup brewing in the kitchen.

I asked to see Dr. Gross. In a few minutes, I was warmly greeted by a beautiful young woman who introduced herself as Mrs. Joy Gross, Dr. Gross' wife. Since I didn't have the strength to carry my luggage, Joy went outside and brought the suitcases in. Then she grabbed the suitcases under one arm and me with the other arm, because I was so weak, and took us all upstairs to a room on the second floor. This was to be my home for a while.

It was a bright, cheery room with two beds. (For the first few weeks I occupied this room, I had it all to myself.) At the time, I really wasn't interested in the physical layout. I was too sick, too weak and had a widespread infection in the bowel, accompanied by a fever. My only desire at the moment was to just drop into bed and stay there, which I did after quickly unpacking.

Perhaps I should explain here that hygienic institutions are *not* fancy, plush spas with matching fancy prices. They are clean, pleasant, and are within reach of the average person's finances. The costs could probably be compared to a stay at an average motel—but in addition you get the doctor's care and attention several times a day, plus his being available 24 hours a day. The food is included when you are eating and you also benefit from the doctor's advice and educational programs concerning your new way of life.

If you compare the cost of a stay at a hygienic institution and the cost of a stay at a general hospital, you will find the cost of one week at the hygienic institution will equal about one day in the general hospital. You will learn and build good health in the hygienic institution, but I doubt if you will in the general hospital (barring emergency care, certain "necessary" surgeries, etc.).

I fell asleep almost immediately, but was awakened soon after by a knock at the door. It was Dr. Gross. He sat on the edge of my bed and we talked for a half-hour or so and he told me that I would be fasting—no food, just water. I was mentally prepared for that, but I didn't know for how long, so I asked him, but he wouldn't commit himself because he really did not know. He told me that each individual is different and each problem is different, so we would take each day as it came. Dr. Gross had an idea of approximately how long he would like me to fast, but, of course, he wouldn't tell me. In our previous little interview he sized me up quite well and knew not to give me a projection too far in advance.

Dr. Gross saw how tired I was and told me to try and get some sleep, after which I was to weigh myself and keep a daily record of my weight changes. When I awoke, I put myself on the scale and recorded 140 pounds in the first page of my diary. I was starting this fast on Thursday, September 3, 1964, at 140 pounds, a 30-pound deficit from my so-called normal weight of 170 pounds (too heavy). I spent a good part of this day sitting outside and getting a little sun. (The first week was spent almost entirely in bed, except for the frequent bowel activity which necessitated me ambulating to the lavatory. Even though I was to abstain from food, except water, for the next six weeks, there was bowel activity every day except for the last few days of the fast. It took about nine or ten days for my body to eliminate the infection and bring down the fever. At no time were any drugs, vitamins, or supplements administered. Everything accomplished was by the body's own ability when left unmolested.) This first fasting day was rather uneventful. No unusual thirst or hunger. Malaise and weakness present. About a dozen B.M.s (diarrhea) with no blood. Slept fair. Short periods of insomnia and restlessness; but not as intense as before coming here. Up twice during the night for B.M.s.

Here follow selections from my diary for the period of my fast and recovery:

Friday, September 4, 1964—Fast, 2nd day: My weight this morning is 139 pounds; a loss of one pound. Sensations of hunger at scattered intervals. Very weak and tired. Some light-headedness on getting up, due to decrease in blood pressure. No headache. No unusual thirst. Six watery B.M.s today and no blood. Feet, legs, and thighs have dull ache. This, coupled with insomnia and restlessness, makes it difficult to fall asleep. Very poor night due to uneasiness plus four or five trips to the lavatory.

Saturday, September 5, 1964—Fast, 3rd day: Coating on tongue, foul breath and taste beginning, as is the thickening of saliva. (This is normal on a fast and occurs in varying degrees, as the body eliminates its wastes or toxic load, which has been accumulating for years. There were many mornings I'd have to take a knife blade and scrape the coating off. I could taste salt, plus many of the drugs coming through the mucous membranes of my mouth. There is nothing known to man that equals the fast as a means of increasing elimination of waste from the blood and tissues.) Weight this morning is 137-½ pounds; a loss of 1-½ pounds from yesterday and a total loss of 2-½ pounds in two days of fasting. No hunger or desire for food, although I can taste certain foods in my mind as I think about them. Very comfortable day. Weakness and tiredness has decreased since yesterday and I feel more alert. Very little thirst. Five B.M.s. today (diarrhea with some blood). Low back (sacral) pain makes it difficult to get from lying to sitting or sitting to standing position, supposedly due to breaking up of calcium deposits in that area, which most people accumulate as age increases. This is quite common and lasts only three or four days, followed by comfort and increased suppleness in the area. Much insomnia and restlessness—very annoying. Blood pressure a little low, but good quality pulses. Must be careful on standing up. If too rapid, lightheaded to almost blackout. Difficult to sleep—restless. Up twice during night for trips to lavatory. Could feel spasms in the large intestine. Blood pressure 118/75.

Sunday, September 6, 1964—Fast, 4th day: Weight this morning 136-½ pounds; a loss of one pound from yesterday and a total loss of 3-½ pounds after three days of fasting. Walking labored. Sense of well-being all day. Light-headed in upright position. Occasional but negligible nausea. No natural hunger or true desire for food. (Usually, sick people like myself have no desire to eat anyway, even though we are forced to as part of medical treatment. The sick body does not have the capacity to properly digest and assimilate or absorb food and this weakens the body further. The fast provides the needed rest for the digestive organs. Now, the average person will experience hunger for about the first three days, after which it subsides and the faster becomes comfortable. I've heard many people state that they tried fasting, couldn't tolerate the hunger, and swore not to fast again. The problem was that they didn't fast beyond three days —they never experienced the most comfortable phase of the fast.) Low back—sacral—pain quite intense when maneuvering into different positions, but most intense when in a bent-over position and trying to straighten up. (Much gas is present most of the time throughout my fast.) Five diarrheal episodes with clot-like material present. Very bad night. Terrible insomnia and restlessness. Not much sleep. Awakened during night for three bouts of diarrhea. (The average person, by this stage of the fast, has ceased to have B.M.s—not true of those with severe, chronic, ulcerative colitis.) Blood pressure 118/78.

Monday, September 7, 1964—Fast, 5th day: Weight 134 pounds; a loss of 2-½ pounds from yesterday and a total loss of six pounds after four days of fasting. Low back pain much eased. Tired, weak, and sluggish, but feel fine mentally and in good spirits. Blood pressure 115/72. Tongue quite coated. Breath and taste very foul. True desire for food absent, but talked much about it and could taste, in my mind, whatever I imagined. Slight increase in thirst, although water is beside me and I drink only when thirsty—never forced. (There is some dehydration when fasting, but depending on the productivity of the fast, our own senses determine how much water is needed. There were some days when a total of two glasses satisfied me and there were other days I used a total of two quarts.) About four poor B.M.s with much gas. Not much sleep—bad insomnia and restlessness. Two trips to lavatory during night.

Friday, September 11, 1964—Fast, 9th day: Weight this morning 128-½ pounds; a loss of ½ pound from yesterday and a total loss of 11-½ pounds after eight days of fasting. Blood pressure 110/68. No headache. (I had no headache the entire length of the fast; however, many people may develop one, especially if they had been drinkers of coffee, tea, alcohol, cola drinks or users of tobacco, condiments, and other indications of "gracious living." There are many crises that may develop during various phases of the fast; headache is just one. Some others are nausea, vomiting, aches, and pains, just to mention a few. Usually the deeper one goes into a fast and the more toxic wastes he eliminates, the more tendency toward various crises, which all come to pass.) Fair day. Insomnia and much intestinal gas during the night.

Sunday, September 13, 1964—Fast, 11th day: Weight 126-½ pounds; a loss of ½ pound from yesterday and a total loss of 13-½ pounds after ten days of fasting. The bowel infection I brought with me has gradually succumbed to the body's defense mechanism—feel better generally and fever is gone. Similar day as yesterday, except my nose and, mainly, my feet have become cold. It is quite annoying and I ask for a hot water bottle. (Cold feet are not uncommon during a fast. Many people experience this phenomenon in one degree or another. My feet remained cold for the remainder of the fast, but the hot water bottle helped a great deal.) Occasional hiccoughs all day.

Monday, September 14, 1964—Fast, 12th day: Weight 126 pounds; a loss of ½ pound from yesterday and a total loss of 14 pounds after 11 days of fasting. Blood pressure 90/64. Not quite as tired, weak, or lethargic. Slight increase in energy. Morale fine, especially when I receive letters from home. Bowel activity all day. Restlessness and insomnia gone, but I sleep only at intervals of several hours or less. (Sleeping became a frustrating problem during the fast, since most of the time is spent resting in bed and napping at intervals all through the day. This made it quite difficult to fall asleep—I was all "slept" out.) I try not to nap during the day and go to sleep as late as possible. I think a lot about my family and how they're getting along. I have their picture on my bedside table.

Tuesday, September 15, 1964—Fast, 13th day: Weight 125-½ pounds; a loss of ½ pound from yesterday and a total loss of 14-½ pounds after 12 days of fasting. Continued bowel activity with much gas formation throughout intestinal tract. Some weakness, but I feel more alert and in good spirits. (I feel much better at this point than when hospitalized 1-½ years ago and forced to eat a high-protein diet three times a day plus a nighttime snack. This was too much food, improperly combined and too difficult for a weakened digestive system to handle. It continued to overwork the colon, which needed the physiologic rest now being given.) No insomnia, but sleep sporadic.

Wednesday, September 16, 1964—Fast, 14th day (2 weeks): Weight 125-¼ pounds; a loss of ¼ pound from yesterday and a total loss of 14-¾ pounds after 13 days of fasting. Several B.M.s. with a mucus, pus-like material containing some blood. Average day, except blood pressure is 84/60. Dr. Gross enters my room and asks me if I am going to fast all day. I stare at him rather surprised, until he laughingly tells me that today is Yom Kippur, the Jewish Day of Atonement. Being Jewish, I have fasted every year on this holiest of days. I have lost track of time here and forgotten about this day, the ironic thing being that I have already been fasting for two weeks. I tell Dr. Gross I am accumulating a 14-year advance reserve for future Yom Kippurs. (As of this writing, at 46 years old, 12 years and many long fasts later, my one-day Yom Kippur fasts are "snaps" because the cleaner the internal environment of the body, the easier the fast. This is why I find it so fascinating and even humorous—my friends and relatives should forgive me—when I observe Jewish people at the end of Yom Kippur day in various throes of agony such as headache, nausea, weakness, dizziness, and even helplessness. A truly healthy individual finds a one-day fast very comfortable and the rest it affords the body very beneficial.)

Thursday, September 17, 1964—Fast, 15th day:

Weight 124-¾ pounds; a loss of ½ of a pound from yesterday and a total loss of 15-¼ pounds after two weeks of fasting. Blood pressure 90/60. Basically same day as yesterday. The days have been sunny and mild, so I've been sitting outside when I'm up to it, occasionally ambling over to the solarium for short periods of sun "au naturel." I'm quite bony now—somewhat resembling a concentration camp inmate, but not quite that bad. It is a rather strange feeling to see myself in the mirror, but as time progresses I shall look worse before I look better. I remind myself of a science fiction movie I once saw entitled "The Incredible Shrinking Man." The subject of food preoccupies our thoughts and conversations, but no true hunger or desire to eat.

Sunday, September 20, 1964—Fast, 18th day: Weight 124 pounds; no loss from yesterday. Blood pressure 90/66. More mentally alert today. Not as tired or weak. Tongue very coated—have been scraping it each morning. Breath and taste are quite foul with much salt coming through tongue and mucous membranes of the mouth. Can't seem to quench thirst. Occasional B.M.s, very foul and consisting of pus-like material. Sporadic sleep.

We are able to fast for long periods of time, particularly while resting, because our bodies live off our stored reserves which we all have in varying degrees. The body has its own wisdom and takes only what it needs from these reserves, no more and no less. Weight loss is also controlled and rationed by this wisdom. Contrary to "popular" belief, the body doesn't go into ketosis or acidosis (a low alkalinity of the blood) from the breakdown of fat, thereby causing death. True, there is some ketosis, but again the body's own innate wisdom keeps this under control. None of these things I've just touched upon happen by chance. None of these things occur haphazardly. There is an order based on natural laws—physiology—whereby our bodies, when left unmolested, automatically and efficiently govern themselves and strive to maintain biochemical balance—homeostasis.

Monday, September 21, 1964—Fast, 19th day: Weight 123-¼ pounds; a loss of ¾ of a pound from yesterday and a total loss of 16-¾ pounds after 18 days of fasting. Blood pressure 94/78. If I include the 30 pound deficit from the illness when I began the fast, then the total weight loss becomes 46-¾ pounds. Thirst decreased. No headache or vomiting and very little nausea or other untoward reaction thus far. Several fetid, pus-like B.M.s. Comfortable day. I experience an amazing phenomenon this 19th fast day: a new surge of energy, no weakness or tiredness, legs have strength with no weakness (previously, walking was slow-motion), can rise from a sitting or lying position without light-headedness and am unusually mentally alert. The more toxic load thrown off by the body, the clearer the mind and all senses become. These last three or four days have been quite a period of detoxification through the pus-like rectal discharges and copious amounts of horrible tasting excretions from the tongue, mucous membranes, and salivary glands.

Tuesday, September 22, 1964—Fast, 20th day: Weight 122-¼ pounds; a loss of 1 pound from yesterday and a total loss of 17-¾ pounds after 19 days of fasting. Very little gas and only one B.M. during the night. No hunger, but my mind is flooded with thoughts of many succulent and delicious foods this entire day and evening, but for some strange reason all through

this fast my mind continues to see, smell, and taste hot
dogs and beans (one of my favorite dishes when I was
a boy). I think of my wife and children each day and
anxiously wait for mail to come from home each day. I
eagerly look forward to several nights during the week
when I allow myself the luxury of a long-distance telephone call so I may talk to my wife and hear her voice.
I also think about my practice and whether or not it is
still afloat, but periodic letters from my good friend, Dr.
Newton Karp, assure me he is keeping it solvent. That
puts my mind at ease because all my expenses are con-
tinuing.

Thursday, September 24, 1964—Fast, 22nd day:
Weight 122 pounds; a loss of ¼ pound from yesterday
and a total loss of 18 pounds after three weeks of fasting.
Blood pressure 88/64 with good pulse quality. Feel wonderful physically, mentally and spiritually, except for a
slight weakness which is understandable at this stage of
the game. Mild light-headedness if I sit or stand up too
quickly. Thick, foul drainage from the sinuses all day,
resulting in the clearest breathing I've had in years. Two
liquid bowel actions today. Dr. Gross checks us in the
morning and again in the late afternoon or early evening.
His home is just a few hundred yards away. I have been
asking him to give me some idea how much longer it
would be until my fast would be broken. (I didn't realize
at the time that the more serious problems usually require
a longer fast. Dr. Gross knew he would prefer a long fast,
if possible, for me. He knew that to break the fast now,
when I'm progressing, would not be in my best interest.
Yet he understood my impatient nature and took me
through the remainder of the fast by degrees and subtle-
ties. In other words, I would ask him when the fast would

be broken and he would say something to the effect that since it's mid-week, let's wait until the weekend. Then when the weekend would roll around, I'd pose the question again and he would give me some logical excuse or reason for fasting a few more days. This is the way he guided me and it helped because psychologically it divided my fast so I would not have to envision long weeks ahead.)

Friday, September 25, 1964—Fast, 23rd day: Weight 121-½ pounds; a loss of ½ pound from yesterday and a total loss of 18-½ pounds after 22 days of fasting. Blood pressure 90/65. Slight fuzziness in the head. One B.M. containing some type of unhealthy tissues from the intestinal tract that the body is finally breaking down and casting out. Very comfortable day, but I don't look forward to the long night ahead, because of being in bed most of the time and taking naps. Furthermore, I find fasting to be one long 24-hour day with no breaks, such as when one is eating three times a day. I stay up late, read a little until the book drops out of my hands, and then try to get to sleep at one o'clock in the morning. Then I wake up wondering how long I have slept, look at my watch and see it is only 10 or 15 minutes later. So I concentrate intently, fall asleep, and wake up thinking the sun will soon be up. But I glance at my watch again and it is perhaps only a half-hour later. This is the battle I fight almost every night during my fast. I'm thankful for my little radio.

Saturday, September 26, 1964—Fast, 24th day: Weight 121-¼ pounds; a loss of ¼ pound from yesterday and a total loss of 18-¾ pounds after 23 days of fasting. Blood pressure 100/60. More salt being excreted through my mouth—causes mild stinging of the tongue.

A wonderfully comfortable day, the only annoying problem being the almost complete dryness of my tongue and mouth with a slight pasty-like mucus. True hunger and desire for food absent. Almost no intestinal gas. Several small, fetid, pus-like rectal discharges. I'm amazed at how fine I feel generally. In fact, this is the best I have felt thus far. I feel as though I could continue the fast indefinitely. The further I get into the fast, the cleaner the mind and body become as deep-seated poisons and wastes are eliminated. This produces profound changes. (From here on I experience unusual clarity of mind, increases in visual acuity, hearing, and smell, greatly increased mental endurance, and an extreme general awareness. For example, I brought with me a variety of crossword puzzles, books, and a chess set. Ideally, one should refrain from anything that taxes any of the senses and burdens the mind during a fast; that also includes television. However, a little occasional light reading does help pass the time. During the early stages of my fast— and even before fasting—I could do a crossword puzzle or two, work out a little problem with my chess set, or read to my tolerance, which would be about 20 to 30 pages. But from this point deep in the fast, until its termination, amazing things happen: as a fairly decent chess player, I now become unbeatable; as a good crossword puzzle solver—but always finding it necessary to use the dictionary for such words as xerus or xat, etc.— I now have instant recall of words that I would ordinarily have to look up in the dictionary; and my mental endurance allows me to read not just double or triple the number of pages I mentioned before, but entire books of 200 to 300 pages without tiring. I don't do these things to set any records; nor do I do them to pass any endurance tests. In fact, I don't make all these things a daily routine because I don't want to jeopardize my chances for a successful fast. I only cite these examples to show some of the marvelous, positive benefits that can accrue from a fast.) The comparative inactivity of the colon at this point is a blessing.

Sunday, September 27, 1964—Fast, 25th day: Weight 120 pounds; a loss of 1-¼ pounds from yesterday and a total loss of 20 pounds after 24 days of fasting. Blood pressure 90/60. Very little gas formation. Several small, liquid B.M.s. I can describe, in one word, the way I feel at this point—healthy! Weak as I am, I can feel health coursing through my body. But within this weakness I feel a tremendous inner strength. It is difficult for me to describe this feeling because one must experience it to understand. Thoughts of food preoccupy my mind. The monotony of routine annoys me. Slept at intervals.

Monday, September 28, 1964—Fast, 26th day: Weight 119-¾ pounds; a loss of ¼ pound from yesterday and a total loss of 20-¼ pounds after 25 days of fasting. As I get deeper into the fast, I find myself having more and more positive thoughts and a feeling of well-being. There seems to be a profound inner calm. Through this experience, so far, I have learned a wonderful self-discipline. Today was similar to yesterday. Missing my family is what bothers me most now. I think of my children often. I think of my wife and the joys we shared together before I became sick. I want very much to be home with them. I feel myself getting better with each passing day. I'm going to make it! There is no doubt in my mind. I actually tremble with anticipation.

Tuesday, September 29, 1964—Fast, 27th day: Weight 120-¼ pounds; a gain of ½ pound from yesterday. I could not believe that after 26 days of fasting and living off my stored reserves there would be a weight gain. It just couldn't be possible. I went to three different scales, but each gave the same reading. My blood pressure today is 96/66. I'm eliminating so much "junk" from my system that the foul taste keeps me on the brink of nausea. In fact, there are times I find it necessary to take a half of a grape and brush it across my tongue to prevent vomiting. At this point, I can taste some of the drugs being eliminated through the mucous membranes of my mouth, the most predominant being phenobarbital. Wide awake and alert. Have been going outside to sit in the sun at intervals. I have incentive. When I perspire, it is not salty. I also notice that if perspiration from my forehead runs into my eyes, there is no stinging or irritation. This evening, Dr. Gross introduced me to a man who had just arrived at the Manor. He had suffered a heart attack six months prior to coming here and his doctors gave him up, but he found out about fasting, etc., and decided to give it a try. The man was afraid to fast. He didn't believe anyone could survive without food for any great length of time and this is why I was introduced to him; so he could see someone who has been fasting for four weeks and is not only alive, but recovering health. This meeting helped him make a decision to fast—and the results were nothing short of fantastic. (In another section I'll mention some of the dramatic cases I observed and followed up over the years, so you can understand the amazing recuperative powers that reside within us if the conditions of health are supplied.)

Thursday, October 1, 1964—Fast, 29th day: Weight 118-¼ pounds; a loss of ½ pound from yesterday and a total loss of 21-¾ pounds after four weeks of fasting. Blood pressure 85/60. Tongue remains heavily coated. Breath and taste extremely foul, almost to the point of nausea, as the body is still eliminating its toxic load. No hunger. Only one B.M. today, which was foul and pus-like. Much belching associated with vague, all-over chest discomfort and discomfort in my neck and throat when I swallow. This is known as a "crisis" of which there can be few or many different types during a fast. Must be careful on rising to a sitting or standing position since light-headedness is yet a factor. (One morning, for example, there came a loud knocking at my door. It awakened me and I jumped right out of bed to answer the door. I blacked out immediately, but before I hit the floor I caromed off the walls like a billiard ball on a table as I fought to stay on my feet. That was one thing I didn't repeat.) This chest discomfort is accompanied by a rather persistent cough. I note this because there is a lessening of muscle control and a weakness of the diaphragm and other muscular units which aid in coughing. This makes coughing quite difficult and is a strange sensation, since it requires great effort and then the cough really does not come out as a cough but as a forced expiration.

Friday, October 2, 1964—Fast, 30th day: Weight 117-¼ pounds; a loss of 1 pound from yesterday and a total loss of 22-¾ pounds after 29 days of fasting. Blood pressure 82/56. The chest, neck and throat discomfort greatly eased, but the weak coughing phase continues. Still have some bowel activity after all this time.

Felt wonderful today. Very alert. Since time weighed heavy, I found several ways to make it pass more quickly. First of all I would think of food, which was on my mind constantly. I was able to close my eyes and visualize many dishes. I could, in these visions, smell and taste them. (I also conjured up some recipes which I thought could be used when I returned home. And you know something? We use these vegetarian recipes at home to this day.) The point of this daydreaming is that time would pass. While I'd mentally concoct these dishes, the hours would slip away. I'd glance at my watch thinking 10 or 15 minutes had elapsed, but in reality it would be an hour or so. Slept poorly. I'd drop off to sleep, awaken and assume I slept for several hours, but when I checked the time it would be maybe 5 minutes or 20 minutes later. This is the way it went for me most of the time.

Saturday, October 3, 1964—Fast, 31st day: Weight 117 pounds; a loss of ¼ pound from yesterday and a total loss of 23 pounds after 30 days of fasting. Blood pressure 102/60. Discomfort in neck and throat when I swallow, which gradually subsides at night. Periodic coughing continues with an occasional sneeze added, but both have a very weak intensity, similar to slow motion. A most unusual experience. Several usual B.M.s. (Another game I played to pass the time and at least break up my day into three parts was called "watch the others eat." It was most successful and satisfying. I would look forward to breakfast, lunch, and supper for those whose fasts had already been broken. Then I would gape at the people eating, watching every bite, every chew, and imagine myself in their place and mentally experience the taste of each piece of luscious fruit or vegetable or whatever they were eating. Then I would sit back, relax, and look forward to the next meal.) Slight fuzziness in my head accompanied by a slight general weakness, but otherwise I feel mentally sharp with a sensation of physical and mental well-being. I feel wonderful and have had a most comfortable day. I have enjoyed most of the evenings because from my window I can watch the sun lower itself beyond the Hudson River, caress the mountainous foothills, and finally slip out of sight, leaving a warm glow hovering in the western sky. Then darkness comes and the sky is ablaze with stars of such magnitude as I had never seen back home where the city lights block out this heavenly artwork.

Sunday, October 4, 1964—Fast, 32nd day: Weight 115-½ pounds; a loss of 1-½ pounds from yesterday and a total loss of 24-½ pounds after 31 days of fasting. Blood pressure 98/58. Mild discomfort in neck and throat, but lessening. At last, no B.M.s today. A most comfortable day. I feel alert and wonderful. Small, multiple warts and other skin blemishes have completely disappeared or are disappearing. All facial pimples are completely gone and have been gone for quite some time. Coughing and sneezing greatly diminished. Just could not lie in bed today; too much pent-up energy and emotion. For the first time in years, I feel alive! I had to get out or I'd bust. In my weakness I feel a tremendous inner strength. Took a slow, slow walk about the grounds. Visited the gymnasium, which was donated by a woman who had fasted here and recovered from arthritis. To one side of the gym was a beautiful flower garden. Further along, I discovered a pond stocked with large goldfish. The water was ice-cold, the pond being spring-fed. The area is heavily wooded and an occasional rabbit goes skittering between the trees. There is a continuous symphony which is given by the wide array of birds by day and crickets, frogs, and owls by night. The majestic Manor house, with its three stories and Ionic-like columns, occupies a central area on the slope of a hill overlooking the mountains and Hudson River in the distance, and giving all viewers a front row seat to the most spectacular sunsets. A short distance away from the main house are the "units," which are six self-contained motel-like rooms for those who might prefer more privacy. The air smells clean and fresh and there is a certain quiet so necessary, so vital, for fasting and obtaining peace of mind.

Monday, October 5, 1964—Fast, 33rd day: Weight 114-¾ pounds; a loss of ¾ of a pound from yesterday and a total loss of 25-¼ pounds after 32 days of fasting. Hurrah! No B.M.s today. Discomfort in chest, neck, and throat gone. Coughing and sneezing stopped. More elimination through mouth causes nausea due to terrible taste. Fleeting sensations of hunger. Usual weakness and tiredness present, but otherwise am alert, sharp, and feel wonderful. Odd sensation to look into the mirror and see what's looking back at me. What happened to that handsome devil that once looked back? One good gust of wind and someone could tie a string on me and have the first human kite. Dry heaves during the night with some bile coming up. Very nauseated. Tiring and exhausting night —so little sleep. Blood pressure 80/50. My skin has marvelous tone, texture, and color.

Tuesday, October 6, 1964—Fast, 34th day: Weight 112-¾ pounds; a loss of two pounds from yesterday and a total loss of 27-¼ pounds after 33 days of fasting. Blood pressure 76/50. No true hunger, but some desire is present. No bowel activity. Slept at intervals. Similar day as yesterday. Few dry heaves with bile, but felt better after. One of the first occurrences on a fast is the diminution of sex drive, with eventual cessation of it. (Interesting to note, however, is that this sex drive is one of the last things to return after the fast is broken, but eventually it returns, and when it does—watch out world! It's likened to putting a high voltage battery in a used car.)

Wednesday, October 7, 1964—Fast, 35th day (5 weeks): Weight 111-¼ pounds; a loss of 1-½ pounds from yesterday and a total loss of 28-¾ pounds after 34 days of fasting. Blood pressure 82/50. No B.M.s. Tongue appears a little clearer. Breath and taste not quite so bad. Feel wonderful and alert. Desire to eat is stronger. I note some amazing changes after five weeks of fasting: Tartar and plaque gone from teeth; gums, which were red and bled easily, are now pink and do not bleed after a vigorous brushing; after six years of severe diarrhea and intestinal spasms, a slight prolapse of the rectum occurred (dropping or sagging of the lower end of the large intestine so that each time a B.M. is tried, a portion of this intestine protrudes through the rectum into the outside world and must be pushed back in). This situation is now corrected—so I suppose one could say the problem with the rectum has been rectified; and, of course, that grapevine of internal and external hemorrhoids are now gone, broken down by the body's own marvelous mechanism. (It's been 12 years since this writing and there have been no recurrences of any of these problems.) Now if this hell-on-earth, this ulcerative colitis could be resolved, this would be truly a miracle—the miracle for which Corinne and I have prayed. I'm hoping, with all

the strength in me, that these benefits from my fast can
be maintained. Only time will tell. (There's still a long,
hard road ahead; but one lesson I shall learn along the
way is that you cannot buy health—you must earn it!)
My fast is supposed to be broken tomorrow and I look
forward to that as much as a child anticipates a Christmas
morning.

Thursday, October 8, 1964—Interruption of fast:
Weight 110 pounds; a loss of 1-¼ pounds from yesterday and a total loss of 30 pounds after 5 weeks of fasting. My anticipation came to an end when a small cup
of clear, freshly made vegetable broth was brought to my
room. Several tablespoons filled me, but I didn't enjoy
it as I had expected. My mouth was still pasty and with
a bad taste. An hour or two later I had several more
tablespoons of the soup and it seemed to bloat me. I
couldn't understand it. (Long fasts are broken very carefully, sometimes with small amounts of diluted, fresh-
squeezed orange juice or small amounts of freshly made
carrot and celery juice or tomato and celery juice. The
particular needs or situations of each individual is taken
into consideration. For example, in my case, citrus wasn't
given because of my past history and Dr. Gross did not
want to take a chance with any fruit acids irritating the
colon. This way, with the broth, I still received some
food value—vitamins, minerals, protein, etc.—and the
broth was very easy on the digestive apparatus. I was
like a newborn infant eating for the first time.) Small
amount of carrot and celery juice added at intervals during the day. Some abdominal cramps and indigestion
throughout the night. Didn't feel well. Much diarrhea and
discomfort. My entire system feels out of whack. I feel
weak all over. Food became repugnant.

Friday, October 9, 1964—Fast, 36th day: Dr. Gross advises me to fast a while longer as my body was not ready to have the fast broken and accept food. Each individual is different and some require a shorter fast, while some are in need of a longer fast. (The body has its own wisdom in letting us know when it's time to break a fast—if we have fasted long enough, that is. A few of the signs are: a genuine return of hunger, clearing of the foul breath, disappearance of the rotten taste with resultant appearance of a sweet taste, and a clearing of the tongue which gradually takes on a clean, pink look.) No weight change. Feel more comfortable not eating at this time.

Sunday, October 11, 1964—Fast, 38th day: Weight 109-¼ pounds; a loss of ½ pound from yesterday and a total loss of 30-¾ pounds after 37 days of fasting. Blood pressure 88/52. Some bowel activity again today. Light-headed and a little weak physically, but resting in bed helps the most. Mentally, very sharp. Have been in a different room for the last few weeks and share it with several men. I've enjoyed this because having people to talk to has helped pass the time. There's an excellent view of the dense wooded area as I lie gazing out the window. I notice the leaves beginning to change colors. Very homesick today, so I telephoned home. Just hearing Corinne's voice was the pick-me-up I needed. She was quite shocked to find out I was still fasting, but understood why after my explanation. She encouraged me to have faith. Never did she discourage me or instill any negative thoughts in my mind. (Sure, things were rough with so little income, her teaching duties, raising the children, and managing everything at home, but we both had an ultimate goal and it was all the experiences we

shared in striving for and attaining that goal that has
brought us as close together as two people can possibly
be.)

Monday, October 12, 1964—Fast, 39th day: Weight
109 pounds; a loss of ¾ of a pound from yesterday and
a total loss of 31 pounds after 38 days of fasting. Blood
pressure 84/56. Light-headedness very prevalent. Most
of the day spent in bed, resting all senses. Bowel action
stopped. I can't really explain it, but there are great
changes taking place. I can feel it. I notice a calmness,
an inner peace which seems almost spiritual. There is no
negativism; only positive thoughts come into mind. I feel
there is nothing I can't do. The word "impossible" does
not exist at this point.

Tuesday, October 13, 1964—Fast, 40th day: Weight
108-¾ pounds; a loss of ¼ pound from yesterday and
a total loss of 31-¼ pounds after 39 days of fasting.
Blood pressure 82/56. Hands, feet, and nose have been
quite cold, but thank goodness for the hot water bottle
which has become a most welcome bed partner. Tongue
very heavily coated. Saliva has become thicker and is
coupled with an extremely rotten taste that causes a
constant nausea, which predisposes to periods of vomiting and dry heaves. Even the rubbing of a squashed
grape across my tongue does not relieve the taste or
nausea. No bowel activity or gas. Strange feeling of well-
being. Slept fairly well.

Wednesday, October 14, 1964—Fast, 41st day:
Weight 108-¾ pounds; no weight loss from yesterday.
Blood pressure 82/56. Water consumption has been varying up to two quarts daily, but never forced and only
when thirsty. Sincere desire for food is more prevalent.

My highly developed senses, mentioned previously, are sometimes annoying. My eyesight has become rated as 20/10, which is better than normal in that I can see at 20 feet what the normal person can see at ten feet. (This of course was not annoying, but the senses of hearing and smell occasionally caused problems: I could perceive the slightest sounds, perhaps a half block or block away, that would continually disturb my rest, such as someone walking down the front steps of a house or walking on gravel or twigs down the road or someone coughing or sneezing or just talking some distance away. The sense of smell was probably the cause of most of the irritations because I could pick up, like a sensitive detection device, noxious odors in the air. I detected car fumes from down the highway, burning of the autumn leaves, which nauseated me, various "stinking" cooking aromas from several homes in the area, and the worst offender of them all—cigarette smoke. I could smell it from people walking down by the highway hundreds of feet away and I knew when someone on the premises was cheating and sneaking a smoke because it would gag me. I would report these incidents of on-the-premises smoking and sure enough Dr. Gross would ferret out the culprit and all hell would break loose.)

Thursday, October 15, 1964—Fast, 42nd and last day (6 weeks): Weight 108-¼ pounds; a loss of ½ pound from yesterday and a total loss of 31-¾ pounds after 41 days of fasting. Blood pressure 90/60. Teeth very pasty. Saliva seems to flow a little freer, but there is so much being eliminated through my mouth now, I find the terrible taste gags me into periodic dry heaves. My impatience to break the fast is wearing on me. I know it is pending. I know how I feel, because even with all that is going on, there is a stronger desire for food. Dr. Gross visits all of us at least twice each day and is usually nearby if needed, since his house is just a few hundred yards away. He came in this afternoon and dropped a subtle hint of a good possibility of breaking the fast tomorrow because of certain signs I was exhibiting. Since those of us who are fasting have extremely foul breath because of the elimination of our toxic loads, I asked Dr. Gross how he could tolerate coming into a room containing three or four of us and breathe the rank air. He laughed and said, "It's perfume." He was serious, because when he detects this "aroma" he knows our bodies are working and one of the little miracles of nature is taking place. The bright, warm autumn day dwindles into evening. I knew I'd have trouble sleeping tonight because of the anticipation of eating tomorrow, so I stayed up quite late, hoping to tire myself enough to fall asleep. I weighed myself before going to bed and found I'd dropped another ¼ pound from this morning (now 108 pounds), making a total loss of 32 pounds after six weeks of fasting. As I glance at myself in the mirror, sans clothes, I can't shake off the sad, but morbidly humorous thought that if Hollywood was to make a movie of the inmates of a German concentration camp, I could get the lead role —no contest!

I had fasted six weeks. It was still rather difficult for me to believe; to believe that weak as I was, I felt better than I had in years. Now the "real" test was coming, but there were yet many hurdles to leap.

CHAPTER VI

Breaking the Fast

I was to remain at the Manor four weeks more to learn how to eat all over again, just as new foods are carefully introduced into the digestive system of a newborn infant until he or she can eat whole foods. For this reason, I'll stay with my diary a while to give you an idea of just such a step-by-step progression.

Friday, October 16, 1964—1st eating day: I know I slept well, because the sun got up long before I did and caressed my face through the window, hinting that I should awaken. The thick, pasty coating on my tongue is almost gone and my tongue is becoming a normal pink color. But the most surprising occurrence is the disappearance of the foul breath and rotten taste, this taste now ranging from neutral to actually fresh and sweet. I have a tremendous desire to eat. It isn't long before Dr. Gross comes scurrying into my room to personally deliver a small bowl of clear vegetable broth and to also feed me the first spoonful because he feels so proud of my accomplishment. This time I enjoy it, allowing the taste to linger a while. That one tablespoonful is a seven-course banquet all rolled into one. The taste is fantastic. (This is the way it is after a fast, whether soup, orange juice, carrot and celery juice, or whatever is used to break the fast. The body is so clean and the taste so unperverted, that the simplest of foods provides a flavor which is indescribable to one who has not fasted. At the time I don't think anything equals it.) I sip the soup very slowly, fighting the temptation to gulp it all down at once. Lunch is another small bowl of the clear vegetable broth. Mid-afternoon I receive four ounces of fresh carrot and celery juice, which I take slowly. Supper is a small bowl of a mixed vegetable soup with some of the vegetables pureed. Later in the evening, about four ounces of fresh carrot and celery juice. A very comfortable day, not only physically but psychologically as well, now that I'm eating. The thrill and enjoyment of eating cannot be expressed in words. Slept a little better.

Saturday, October 17, 1964—2nd eating day: Wake up feeling alive and vital for the first time. My tongue is completely pink and smooth. Weight 110-¾ pounds; a gain of 2-¾ pounds after one day of eating. Blood pressure 86/60. Very hungry. Breakfast: pureed zucchini squash soup. Lunch: two very ripe bananas, mashed. Mid-afternoon snack: cup of pureed tomato-vegetable soup. Supper: four ounces of carrot and celery juice and a mashed banana. (All foods eaten, with the exception of a dry, no-salt, no-chemicals-added cottage cheese, are fresh natural foods grown from the ground, unadulterated, unprocessed, and unchemicalized. Nothing is canned or bottled. This includes all fruits, vegetables, nuts, and seeds. The nuts and seeds—pumpkin or sunflower—are unsalted and unroasted. The diet is vegetarian and no meat is ever used. I'll explain all this in a subsequent chapter.) The way my fast is being broken is not necessarily the way someone else might have their fast broken, because each person is an individual and has different needs and idiosyncracies. Many fasts are broken on such things as orange juice, carrot and celery juice, and various vegetable juices. My situation is rather unique in that I have been forbidden by my past doctors to eat anything with roughage. It has been over six years since I've had any of this type of food. The purpose of this fast is to allow healing so this type of food may be eaten and handled by the body. Had five B.M.s of varying looseness between 6 p.m. and 10 p.m.

Sunday, October 18, 1964—3rd eating day: Wake up hungry and feeling strong and alert. Able to arise from any position without light-headedness. Weight 112-½ pounds; a gain of 1-¾ pounds from yesterday and a total gain of 4-½ pounds after two days of eating. Blood pressure 90/60. It is a delight to awaken with a relish for food and to look forward to the rest of the day. Breakfast: two baked apples. A semi-formed B.M. after breakfast. Lunch: pureed tomato-vegetable soup, small cup of dry cottage cheese. (Nuts—ground at this stage—would be preferable, but because of the severe damage to my large intestine, Dr. Gross was being very conservative at the beginning. Eventually, miracle of miracles, I shall be able to properly digest nuts as a source of concentrated protein.) A semi-loose B.M. after lunch. Feel marvelous today. Able to take a longer walk. Tremendous feeling of energy and well-being. Not bothered by gas in stomach or intestines all day. This is the first time in the six years of medical treatment I am "gas-free." Supper: blended, steamed acorn squash and a baked potato. A B.M. after supper and again at 10:00 p.m. (The cycle of peristalsis

—intestinal motility—is still very much stimulated by the intake of food. This gradually lessens, although in my case it will take several years; but I'm patient. After all, what else have I to do but regain health? Nothing else matters without it.) Sleep was at intervals, but improved.

Tuesday, October 20, 1964—5th eating day: Weight 115-¾ pounds; a gain of 1-¾ pounds from yesterday and a total gain of 7-¾ pounds after four days of eating. Breakfast: four baked apples and a mashed banana. Lunch: pureed steamed peas and two baked potatoes. Supper: pureed steamed asparagus, pureed steamed carrots, and two baked sweet potatoes (yams). Some indigestion present all evening. Six B.M.s today, with some mass to them, usually following after each meal. Spent most of the day resting in bed. I take occasional walks, but enjoy most talking with the people here. They are from all walks of life, religions, and races. We all have one thing in common and that is we are all sick in one degree or another and are trying to regain our most precious possession—health. Of course there are many people who have good health who come here periodically to fast, rest, re-charge their batteries, so to speak, and maintain their health. But even with all this camaraderie, I wish more than ever to be home. I've spent most of the last few weeks resting in bed. I've watched summer pass, the leaves change into glorious splashes of color and then say goodbye to their summer home in the trees as they flutter to the ground. Autumn is in the air and the days are mild, but the mornings and evenings are crisp. I love to take walks now that the leaves are fallen. I love the sound of brittle leaves crunching deliciously beneath my feet, although it makes me more homesick as I'm reminded of the long walks Corinne and I take in autumn. Sleep is sporadic, but deepest in the early morning hours.

Wednesday, October 21, 1964—6th eating day: Weight 117-¾ pounds; a gain of 2 pounds from yesterday and a total gain of 9-¾ pounds after five days of eating. Blood pressure 96/60. Breakfast: four baked apples and four mashed bananas. Lunch: pureed vegetable stew, pureed steamed green beans, and two baked potatoes. Supper: pureed mixed vegetables and two baked potatoes. Three B.M.s today with more mass and less looseness. Wonderful day. I continue to feel vital, alive, and gaining in strength. I anticipate and relish each meal and each morsel of food with a zest I have never known before. It is a sensation I wish never to abandon or to have abandon me. Slept fairly. Up only once for trip to the "john," whereas in the past years I would wake at least five or six times a night to heed the urge. In fact, ulcerative colitis victims are usually annoyed most during the night, because the cramping and spasms constantly cause them to waken. But in the morning as soon as they are awake, the slightest movement, because the colon is like a straight tube, causes repeated and hectic journeys to the bathroom until there is nothing left to evacuate. This just adds to the already depressing, enervating, and sometimes disgusting state of "existence" in which we seem to be hopelessly suspended.

Thursday, October 22, 1964—7th eating day: Weight 121-¼ pounds; a gain of 3-½ pounds from yesterday and a total gain of 13-¼ pounds after six days of eating. Breakfast: eight baked apples and five bananas. (This is the most I have eaten for breakfast at Pawling. This is actually too much food, particularly for one who doesn't need excessive stimulation of the intestinal tract, but in my case the appetite became ravenous and had to be satisfied or I'd have become very nervous and tense. This only lasted about two weeks and then tapered off to a point where I needed only surprisingly small amounts of food to satisfy the body's requirements. This ravenous appetite has occurred on all my subsequent fasts because, as you can see by the rapid weight gains, I'm a fast rebounder and am able to utilize all my food. During the years of active ulcerative colitis, I had a malabsorption problem, as most of those afflicted do, and whatever I ate would pass hurriedly through me and out again, many times unchanged and looking the same as it did when I put it in my mouth. So what happens over the years? Even though we colitis victims eat, we suffer from malnutrition because we don't digest and assimilate (absorb and utilize) the food. There were times when I ate so much at the Manor that Dr. Gross actually ran out of food and had to dash to the market immediately so the other people could eat.) Lunch: extra large bowl of pureed steamed celery and three baked potatoes. Supper: large bowl of pureed steamed green beans, large bowl of pureed zucchini squash, and two baked potatoes. Five, you should pardon the description, semi-formed and mushy B.M.s today. A very comfortable and enjoyable day.

Friday, October 23, 1964—8th eating day: Weight 122-¾ pounds; a gain of 1-½ pounds from yesterday and a total gain of 14-¾ pounds after one week of eating. Blood pressure 98/60. Breakfast: two baked apples and, would you believe it, six bananas. Lunch: bowl of pureed steamed celery and two bowls of mashed baked potatoes and mashed steamed carrots (about five carrots and three potatoes). Supper: large bowl of pureed steamed peas, a whole avocado, and a small bowl of pureed brown rice. Comfortable day. Six "mix and match" B.M.s today. The "skeleton" appearance is gone and my face is pretty well filled in. It's a pleasure to peek in the mirror now and see that handsome devil returning.

Sunday, October 25, 1964—10th eating day: Weight 124-¾ pounds; a gain of ½ pound from yesterday and a total gain of 16-¾ pounds after nine days of eating. Blood pressure 100/70. Breakfast: four baked apples followered a little later by a bowl of dry cottage cheese. Lunch: pureed steamed cauliflower, pureed steamed celery and carrots, and three baked potatoes. Supper: pureed steamed celery, pureed steamed butternut squash, and two baked potatoes. Exercised lightly in the gym. I plan to do this on alternate days. I take walks to my tolerance and at no time do I tax myself. Most of the time is still spent resting in bed. Four semi-loose B.M.s today. What a blessing compared to the 20 to 30 B.M.s a day in the latter stages of the illness, even while under medical care and being dosed and poisoned with so many drugs.

Tuesday, October 27, 1964—12th eating day: Weight 125-½ pounds; a gain of ¼ pound from yesterday and a total gain of 17-½ pounds after 11 days of eating. Blood pressure 110/66. Breakfast: seven baked apples followed by a little later by a bowl of dry cottage cheese. Lunch: pureed steamed cauliflower, pureed mixed vegetables, pureed steamed peas, and two baked potatoes. Supper: my first attempt at a meal with no purees, except for the raw salad. Pureed, raw, mixed vegetable salad (romaine lettuce, carrots, cucumber, celery, green pepper, and tomato), steamed peas, steamed carrots and cel-

ery, and two steamed potatoes. Ten B.M.s during the day
and several during the night. (Despite these many B.M.s,
I am absorbing nutrition from the food and putting on
healthy weight.)

Thursday, October 29, 1964—14th eating day: History was made this morning! I had my first formed B.M.
in six years. This may sound strange to those who have
never had ulcerative colitis, but I laughed and cried at
the same time. I could not believe it. I think I was as
proud as the father of a newborn infant. I called Dr.
Gross and gave him the news. I also announced the event
to some of my friends at the Manor and then I called
home and told my wife. In fact, I was so elated that if I
had a camera, I probably would have taken a photograph
of "it" for posterity. (The importance of this was the fact
that I was getting better, evolving health. True, this was
not going to be a regular occurrence in these early years,
but it was an indication of things to come—and they
surely did.) Weight 126-½ pounds; a gain of ½ pound
from yesterday and a total gain of 18-½ pounds after 13
days of eating. Breakfast: six baked apples and three
whole bananas. Lunch: vegetable soup (zucchini squash,
tomato, celery, carrots, corn, green beans, and peas),
steamed carrots and artichokes, bowl of natural (whole
grain or brown) rice. Supper: pureed raw vegetable
salad, steamed beets with the tops (the tops are very rich
in amino acids, the protein building blocks), three
steamed potatoes. So far, I seem to be tolerating the
change toward increased roughage. I have not noticed
any digestive disturbance or bowel irritation, except an
occasional but decreasing incidence of indigestion since
the introduction of the pureed raw salads. Eight semi-

formed B.M.s, the greatest frequency occurring at night.

For the next few days the routine was similar, the ultimate goal being a basically raw vegetarian diet—live foods; a diet my past doctors, particularly Dr. Kale, said I would never be able to eat. These days have been very comfortable and I feel wonderfully alive, much stronger, and have an anticipation and relish for simple plain vegetarian fare. I feel little or no discomfort or spasms, which is the first time in the six years of this disease, regardless of past hospitalizations, drugs, treatments, etc.

I notice very little need for water now. Sometimes go several days without it. This is due to the abundance of water contained in the raw fruits and vegetables. In fact, the less cooked food, the avoidance of condiments, and overeating, then the less is the actual thirst for water. Of course vigorous physical exertion will increase the body's need for water.

Sunday, November 1, 1964—17th eating day: Today started out uneventfully, but it was to be a special day for me—a milestone. I was to have my first raw, whole vegetable salad in six years. It was to be at supper. I remember Dr. Kale forbidding me to eat roughage because of the potential devastating effects to a damaged, debilitated colon. I was frightened. I didn't know how much healing had taken place or if I could tolerate this roughage without serious consequences. However, the body does have extraordinary healing power when it is given the proper circumstances, which it had been given here at the Manor. Nevertheless, I spent most of the day anticipating eating that salad at supper. By the time supper was ready, I was running a fever of 100° and trembling because of the built-up anxiety. Dr. Gross personally brought in the salad and said he was honored to serve it to me because whatever had been accomplished this far, I had earned. The salad was in a small bowl and consisted of romaine lettuce, celery, cucumber, and shredded carrots. Dr. Gross instructed me to "take an hour to eat it." This was to be the first step in a more natural, raw diet. I did take an hour to eat that salad and then I sat back and waited for something to happen. To my surprise there was no explosion, no violent reaction. In fact, I felt comfortable. There was some indigestion during the night, but I had not eaten raw food in six years. (This indigestion occurred for the next couple of days and then subsided and did not recur.)

Thursday, November 5, 1964—21st eating day: Weight 131-¼ pounds; a gain of 2-¾ pounds from yesterday and a total gain of 23-¼ pounds after 20 days of eating. Blood pressure 110/66. Took a short, early morning jog and felt marvelous. I've been waking up at 6:00 a.m. feeling refreshed, rested, and raring to go. I feel alive and vital. Breakfast: four oranges and about four ounces of raw peanuts ground to a nut butter. Lunch: a half of a honeydew melon, two pears, three bananas, and a few dates. Supper: large raw vegetable salad, steamed asparagus, and eggplant parmigiana stew. I notice an increased endurance in my reading ability—speed, concentration, etc. Visual and auditory acuity increased.

Friday, November 6, 1964—22nd eating day: Weight 134-¼ pounds; a gain of 3 pounds from yesterday and a total gain of 26-¼ pounds after three weeks of eating. I'm anxious to go home. I'm ready to get back into the normal routine of life—to work, to play, to be with Corinne and my children, and to live again. Dr. Gross estimates a few more days here, just to see how I'll be handling the diet change toward the increased roughage. Breakfast: one whole grapefruit, two oranges, and four ounces of filbert nuts ground fine. Lunch: a half of a honeydew melon, one persimmon, grapes, and two bananas. Supper: large raw vegetable salad, steamed broccoli, and a bowl of whole grain rice. I have not had any desire to eat meat, nor have I had a desire for alcohol, tea, coffee, chocolate, tobacco, white bread, salt, white sugar and its products, processed and denatured foods, or anything else that breeds ill health. These things have, fortunately, been eliminated from my life, just as have all the drugs that were poisoning my system for so long.

Saturday, November 7, 1964—23rd eating day: Weight 134-¾; a gain of ½ pound from yesterday and a total gain of 26-¾ pounds after 22 days of eating. Blood pressure 110/70. Breakfast: three oranges and four ounces ground, raw peanuts. Lunch: a quarter of a watermelon, grapes, apple, and strawberries. Supper: large raw vegetable salad, steamed peas, and two baked potatoes. During the past week or so, Dr. Gross has been taking me along for the ride on some of his daily errands. I've enjoyed getting out and seeing the beautiful countryside with the Hudson River ever in the distance. I look forward to these outings. We visited various historic places, but today was special. We visited the Roosevelt estate about nine miles toward the southern end of Hyde Park. I was even so bold as to pick a small bag of apples from the orchard.

Sunday, November 8, 1964—24th eating day: Weight 135 pounds; a gain of ¼ pound from yesterday and a total gain of 27 pounds after 23 days of eating. Breakfast: two grapefruits, three oranges, and four ounces of ground almonds (still quite a volume of food, but it soon begins to taper off). Lunch: grapes, two apples, one banana, and one avocado. Supper: large raw vegetable salad, steamed celery and peas, and one acorn squash. (I know the subject of B.M.s has been brought up throughout the book and it is hardly an exciting topic, but it is important since it bears a relationship to the return of normal function and healing of the large intestine, which medical opinion said could not regenerate. So periodically, if you will, I'll give you progress reports on this part of my life.) Bowel activity varies at this point from one or two to six or eight per 24 hour day and ranges from some looseness to semi-formed and formed. Another interesting occurrence is the fact that celery, corn, etc., does not show up in the stools as undigested. When I had the active ulcerative colitis, many pieces of roughage foods would appear. This also occurs in so-called healthy individuals I've questioned. This only proves that not only has healing taken place, but function and strength in the intestinal tract has developed through the body's own ability.

Monday, November 9, 1964—25th eating day: Weight 135-¼ pounds; a gain of ¼ pound from yesterday and a total gain of 27-¼ pounds after 24 days of eating. Dr. Gross informed me this morning that I can plan on going home in a few days. I waste no time in making a decision to leave on Friday the 13th, just four days from today. I know the days will not pass fast enough now. Breakfast: one grapefruit, two oranges, and four ounces ground, raw cashews. Lunch: a chunk of watermelon, slice of cantaloupe, two apples, four peaches, and several dates. Supper:

large raw vegetable salad, steamed zucchini squash, and two steamed potatoes. I notice the stools are not as foul as they were when I was so ill and when I ate meat. In fact, foul stools are characteristic of meat eaters because of the meat's putrefaction in the intestinal tract; while in vegetarians—particularly those who eat a predominantly raw diet—the stools are virtually odorless for the most part, indicating no toxic elements in the colon. (I beg your indulgence for this additional bit on bowels.)

Tuesday, November 10, 1964—26th eating day: Weight 136-¼ pounds; a gain of 1 pound from yesterday and a total gain of 28-¼ pounds after 25 days of eating. Worked out a bit more vigorously in the gym this morning, followed by 30 minutes of cross-country jogging. (I was a cross-country runner in college and it was an exhilarating sensation to be able to get back in the groove.) Breakfast: three oranges and four ounces of ground cashews. Lunch: half a cantaloupe, one plum, blueberries, and dates. Supper: large raw vegetable salad, vegetable stew, and a bowl of whole grain rice. I thought of the many friends I had made in the two and one-half months I've been here and of some of the dramatic recoveries I witnessed. I am awed by the inherent and miraculous ability of the body to heal itself when it is left alone.

Wednesday, November 11, 1964—27th eating day: Weight 136-½ pounds; a gain of ¼ pound from yesterday and a total gain of 28-½ pounds after 26 days of eating. Blood pressure 110/74. Woke up at 6:00 a.m. full of energy. It's still a novelty to me to be able to wake up in the morning and actually look forward to each day and to life rather than to dread each day, to suffer physically, mentally, and emotionally and to wish for death.

Took a light two-mile cross-country jog this morning. Breakfast: one grapefruit, two oranges and three to four ounces of whole peanuts. (From here on, the nuts and sunflower seeds, etc., are no longer ground. The teeth will do the work. The building up to these whole foods has been very gradual, but it was necessary to accustom the rejuvenated intestinal tract to the foods it was meant to handle. There are times when at home we make our own peanut butter because my boys love it and it's so superior to the store-bought, roasted-out, and adulterated mess. Once you eat homemade raw peanut butter, you just can't go back to the commercial stuff.) Lunch: large raw vegetable salad, steamed yellow summer squash, and two steamed potatoes. Supper: vegetable soup, large raw vegetable salad, steamed green beans, and a bowl of whole grain rice. Slept much better.

Thursday, November 12, 1964—28th eating day: Weight 137 pounds; a gain of ½ pound from yesterday and a total gain of 29 pounds after 27 days of eating. Blood pressure 112/74. Breakfast: two whole grapefruit and about four ounces of filbert nuts. Lunch: strawberries, grapes, apple, and a whole avocado. Supper: large raw vegetable salad, bowl of steamed peas, asparagus, green beans, and a buckwheat groats (kasha) casserole. I get a little nervous when I think of leaving tomorrow. I've been here two and one-half months now and it's as if I've always lived here. (Over the ensuing years, Pawling Manor *does* become a home away from home.) I spent part of the day thinking back, all the way back, to the year 1958 when I first became ill. I relived that six-year nightmare under medical care, the transition period when Natural Hygiene was presented to me, and then the entire magnificent experience here—the six-week fast, the careful and methodical breaking of the fast, with the eventual attainment of the goal to be able to eat a basically raw vegetarian diet after the body had healed itself—something my doctors said was impossible. It's so difficult to believe what I've been through and that this first phase of my rebirth (?) has passed. (One thing I've learned over these past 12 years is that whether it is good, bad or indifferent, "everything comes to pass.") Not much sleep. Too many thoughts of home, my wife, children, my practice, and a myriad of other important and even nonsensical items.

Friday, November 13, 1964—29th eating day: Weight 137-½ pounds; a gain of ½ pound from yesterday and a total gain of 29-½ pounds after four weeks of eating. Blood pressure 112/74. Breakfast: two oranges and about four ounces of whole almonds. Lunch: romaine lettuce and celery, one pear, one apple, a dish of dates, and figs. Supper: large raw vegetable salad, steamed butternut squash, and a special treat since I would be leaving this evening; Mrs. Gross (Joy) made what was to be one of my favorite fancy vegetarian dishes in the future—eggplant parmigiana (broiled eggplant, mushrooms, onions, green pepper, tomatoes, etc., topped with mozzarella cheese).

This was a very emotional day for me. This was the day for which I had been planning and waiting, yet as much as I wanted to go home I had a desire to remain here. I must assume it was the security and dependency of being here and I knew this umbilical cord must be severed so I could be my own man again. I had learned a great deal from Dr. Gross about Natural Hygiene and myself, and I had enough knowledge of natural living to carry me through my day-to-day living when I returned to the proverbial rat race.

Part of the day was spent packing and saying good-byes to the many friends I had made in the past two and one-half months. I took a long walk through the country-side. I wanted to be alone, to think. The mid-November air was a bit chilly, but I didn't mind. It was great to be alive, to have health, and to be in one piece. The way I was feeling then, there could have been rain, snow, or sleet and it wouldn't have made any difference. When you have health, you can cope with anything and there's nothing you can't do when there's a positive determination. When you are ill, everything tends toward nega-tivism; but when you have vibrant health, you exude an aura of positiveness. You become positive in body, mind, emotion, and spirit.

Dr. Gross came to my room about 6:00 p.m. and had a last minute chat with me. (My train was scheduled to depart from Rhinecliff, six miles away, at 8:00 p.m.) He advised me to get right back into the swing of things when I returned home. I was to return to Pawling Manor next year and for succeeding years for subsequent fasts until I reach a maximum of healing and a high level of health. Right now I would say I'm 50 percent to 60 per-cent better than when I first came here. It took many years to evolve disease and it would take a number of years to undo all the wrongs and evolve good health. There is no instant cure. Many people spend most of their lives and money seeking it, though; but it is not to be. You just cannot buy good health—you must earn it. You must work at it and build it; but it takes time, a little self-discipline, a little knowledge and understanding of the basic principles of natural living, and sometimes a perserverance that is unshakeable. There is no other investment one can make that will pay dividends as high. Dr. Gross also suggested I fast one or two days per week, say like Monday and Thursday. I was to keep in touch to report my progress or any problems as the need arises. (I have developed a rapport and a kinship with Bob and Joy Gross that will not only endure but will deepen as the years pass.) Time for leaving was almost here and Bob insisted he drive me to Rhinecliff to catch my train. This time I carried my own luggage; not like when I first arrived here and Joy had to carry my luggage and support me at the same time. Bob stayed with me, giving me some personal and confidential bits of advice until the train arrived. Bob and I shook hands. My eyes were beginning to tear and I couldn't say much. I didn't want to get emotional, but it was showing. I could only utter a simple, "Thank You!" Then I boarded the train.

I had taken a roomette again because I did enjoy the privacy and thought I might be able to get a good rest. The trip would take about 13 hours. I would arrive in Detroit at 9:00 a.m. I settled back and tried to keep my mind blank as I stared out the window into the night, but it was impossible. I tried reading and couldn't. Too many random thoughts darted in and out of my mind; thoughts of what *was,* what *is,* and what might be. I also had mixed emotions; I was depressed yet elated. But the closer I got to home, the more elation I felt.

A few hours later I felt hungry, so I reached for the snack bag Joy had given me. It was totally unlike the "last supper" I brought with me two and one-half months ago. This time there was a luscious variety of fresh fruit.

It was after midnight when I pulled down the bed, jumped in, and tried to fall asleep. But my mind was so active I couldn't sleep, so I just looked out the window and watched the little towns pass in the night. I finally did get to sleep but it was a very sporadic sleep, the kind that leaves you groggy when you get up in the morning.

I awoke about 6:00 a.m. and couldn't fall back to sleep. Too much anxiety. The same type of anxiety I experienced upon returning to the United States with the army after a tour of duty in Korea; a butterflies-in-the-stomach feeling. But soon the feeling eased as my eyes caught a glimpse of the sun peeking up over the horizon in the southeastern sky and I watched its glow illuminate the countryside.

(I didn't know it at this time—Corinne admitted to me years later—but she had a great fear of my returning. She was afraid of how I would look. This unknown factor kept her in a slightly tense state, but I had filled out enough to be able to pass for any human being.)

It wasn't long before the conductor came through and called off Detroit as the next stop. I gathered my luggage and moved to the front of the car. The train eased its way into the railroad yard and finally came to a stop in the station.

I juggled all my belongings, stepped off the train, and made my way hurriedly toward the gates inside the depot. I paused momentarily at the big iron gates, my heart pounding fiercely, and then stepped through into the beginning of a new life.

CHAPTER VII

A Return to Life

At the far end of the depot I could see my father, my four-year-old son, and my wife. I was half walking and half running until I finally reached them. Corinne and my son, Irwin, stared at me for a few seconds and then we all embraced. It was good to be home.

I felt Corinne studying me and she could hardly believe the amazing physical transformation that had taken place. So it was for this reason, right here in the train station, that my wife made a vow to change our way of living. We would follow Natural Hygiene in all of its tenets and we would raise our two boys as vegetarians.

During the drive home, Corinne told me my mother was staying with our other son, Darryl, who was 11 months old. Looking out the car window, I saw a sunny Saturday and was grateful for the weekend I'd spend at home before jumping right back into my normal routine on Monday. Irwin continued to look at me as we drove, and Corinne whispered to me that he was waiting for me to tell him how big he had grown since I went away. I suppose I didn't make enough fuss over him at the depot, so I acknowledged the fact that he had grown so tall, and he beamed satisfactorily.

After arriving home, we talked of my experiences for hours, of the people I met, and some of their amazing cases of recovery under natural living—many of whom were given up by their doctors, as in my case. Corinne still couldn't believe the way I looked. She said it was as if I had been reborn; and the truth of the matter is that I really felt reborn. This was probably the motivating force in her strong determination to change our way of life as soon as possible to one that would assure the attainment of health.

Corinne was already formulating plans to depart from our so-called "normal" or "conventional" way of living. Since Natural Hygiene requires a certain degree of self-discipline, some sacrifice, if you will, and almost seems to go against most things we've been led to believe are correct or true, many people can't make this change overnight and require a gradual transition period. But Corinne was able to do this at once because she accepted the fact and knew that it was right. She began by eliminating all meat from our home. Then she went through the cupboards and threw out the items that were harmful to the body or had no place in proper nutrition, such as canned foods, processed foods, anything containing food additives, coffee, tea, alcohol, tobacco, salt, white sugar and its products, white flour and any of its products, chocolate, soda pop, candy, potato chips, and all other junk foods.

This cleaning accomplished, we went to the market and purchased enough fresh produce to stock our two refrigerators. There was an abundance of raw, fresh fruits and vegetables. We went to a health food store and purchased a variety of raw nuts (peanuts, cashews, pecans, almonds, filberts, Brazil nuts), seeds (pumpkin and sun-flower) and such dried fruits as raisins, figs, and dates. The reason we used the health food store was that the nuts and seeds (our source of concentrated protein) are raw, unsalted, and unadulterated; the dried fruits are sun-dried, unsprayed, unsulfured, and poison-free.

By Monday morning, our family was ready to begin its adventure into Natural Hygiene (natural living). Breakfast for Corinne, Irwin, and me consisted of fresh grapefruit, oranges, and nuts, while little Darryl had to be maintained on an infant-type diet, although he was alternated on raw, unpasteurized goat milk, fresh fruit and vegetable juices, and pureed fruits and vegetables. You could call it baby food, but it wasn't commercially adulterated. We made it fresh and pure each meal. The goat milk had been used after Corinne stopped nursing Darryl. If possible, every mother has an obligation to nurse her child to give it a proper start in life and I feel it negligent if she does not nurse for reasons of vanity. Nursing is as natural as breathing and gives the infant marvelous benefits that cannot be gotten from chemical formulas, which do not supply the infant's needs of life or allow it to attain optimum health. Today's pasteurized cows' milk is no better and really has no place in the human diet after the teeth have erupted. Only the human continues to drink milk after weaning.

My family loved their breakfast and was looking for-ward to lunch, which was a fresh fruit plate with a variety of fruits to select, such as apples, bananas, berries, melons, pears, grapes, dates, and peaches (which were still available). Supper was also anticipated, which con-sisted of a huge raw vegetable salad (romaine lettuce, celery, carrots, cucumber, green pepper, cabbage, and cauliflower). The salad was pureed for Darryl. We also had a steamed vegetable (green beans) and a brown rice casserole. The meals were very simple and I've never seen my wife and children enjoy eating as much as they did on that first day. However, the meals were only a sample of how and what we eat and are not to be construed as the be-all and end-all of our existence. A later chapter will cover, in more detail, the how, what, and why of the vegetarian diet and its rationale.

Coincidental as it may seem, my older son Irwin, who had been living "conventionally," had developed so-called allergies over the past six months or so. He was sneezing, coughing, wheezing, and his nose and eyes were ever "running" and itching terribly. He was just under four years old, but we saw personality changes taking place due to his constant irritation and suffering. The doctor who examined him, just before I went away, said Irwin was suffering from allergies and would need some 150 patch tests made on his back (which we wouldn't allow) and then he would be required to take drugs perhaps the rest of his life to "control" the symptoms. We were also instructed to get rid of the wool blankets, the feather pillows, the dust on the floor, and, last but not least, our two cats which had been in our household for years. Nothing was mentioned about diet by the doctor, who considered it vaguely relevant to health.

Within several weeks on the vegetarian program, eating most of the foods raw or unfired and avoiding the items mentioned a few pages back, all of Irwin's symptoms began lessening until they had completely disappeared two or three months later. (It is 12 years later as of this writing and we still have cats, wool, feather pillows and dust—forgive me, Corinne—however, Irwin has had no recurrence.)

We have watched both our boys grow and thrive on a properly handled vegetarian diet with periodic short fasts. Their physical and mental development has been a beautiful thing to watch. (In this year of 1976, Irwin will be 16 years old and Darryl will be 13 years old.) We have raised them virtually free of disease. Irwin was almost four years old when we entered Natural Hygiene, so he did have a vaccination, but has had no inoculations since. Darryl has had one vaccination. Both boys, early in our transitional stage, did contract one of the childhood diseases. But up to the present time, they have had no childhood diseases, as their natural resistance and immunity has been built to function at a peak as a result of nourishing their bodies with live foods.

Neither boy has any dental caries (cavities) and they don't drink fluoridated water or use fluoridated toothpaste. Oh yes, we've been told by many people that heredity plays a big role. Well, if heredity played such a big role, both our boys would have cavities in every tooth in their mouths. Proper diet! Yes, proper diet is the key, particularly begun right from birth and even ideally begun in the prospective parents.

This reminds me of an incident that occurred with my dentist. Over the years, as my mouth became a silver mine, he remarked about my poor dental health. There was much tartar and plaque deposited on the teeth, while the gums were an unhealthy dark red and bled quite easily and freely at the slightest touch of a toothbrush. However, several months after returning from my first fast, I went in for a check-up and the dentist was amazed at the remarkable changes that had taken place. (He talks about it to this day.) Tartar and plaque were completely gone and the gums exhibited a healthy pink color and did not bleed easily, a fact I demonstrated by scraping a dry bristle toothbrush across my gums.

Six months after my return home, I decided to pay a visit to Dr. Kale. My weight had leveled off at about 160 pounds, my blood pressure had stabilized at between 115/75 to 120/80 (where it has remained all these years) and I must say I looked great. Upon entering Dr. Kales's reception room, I was warmly greeted and ushered into his private office by the nurse. A short time later, Dr. Kale entered and we shook hands as he volunteered how marvelous I looked. He sat down, propped up his feet and asked me to tell him "all about it." He listened attentively as I related the entire experience. When I finished, he sat back, glanced up at the ceiling, and with a slight air of medical haughtiness, told me it was psychological, that I was probably going to have a remission anyway, and that mentally I knew something was being done so I got better. He just couldn't conceive of the idea that the body has a tremendous capacity to heal itself when given the proper circumstances. (Animals have been fasting since they have inhabited our planet.) So I posed a question to Dr. Kale. I asked him to recall the time when he hospitalized me for five weeks. He remembered. I told him that all the while I was in the hospital being "treated," I knew something was being done. So why did I get worse? I am still waiting for the answer.

Dr. Kale then tried to convince me I was living abnormally. So I told him I was thriving on the very foods he said I could never eat and I asked him if he ate vegetables. He said he did and I told him he probably eats most of them cooked or canned. Then I asked him if he ate fruit and he said he did. I told him he probably doesn't eat an abundance and that much of it is canned. Finally I asked if he ate nuts and seeds and he said yes, but I told him that what he ate were salted and roasted (dead—cremated, if you will), so all-in-all I was living not too differently. But he disagreed and stated that most people would rather have the operation (cutting out the large bowel and rectum, with the portable toilet opening out of the abdomen) so they could live "normally," eat whatever they desired, and enjoy life. *Enjoy life? How?* He completely missed the point, the rationale, and the purpose of a way of life that not only allows the body the chance to recuperate—regardless of what disease it has—but allows the body to evolve such a vital health that disease is virtually prevented. It cannot be refuted that it is better to prevent than to try to cure.

I left Dr. Kale's office quite disappointed, but I remembered my own situation not too long ago when I also closed my mind to this because it didn't jibe with my medical training. The mind is like a parachute—it only functions when open.

(Over the years, I've asked hundreds of people that if they were confronted with the two choices of doing what I have done and living as I am now or having that radical and drastic surgery so they could live "normally," what would be their choice? I have yet to hear anyone state they would have the surgery first before giving Natural Hygiene a try.)

For the next six months, I was busy returning to the normal activities of my life. I was practicing podiatry full time, although my practice had to be built up again. (In fact, it became frustrating for me to build up my practice each time I went away for these long fasts, but it was necessary and I just made up my mind to hang in and the hell with anything else.) Our family life became enjoyable and what made for an even closer relationship was our common bond—the attainment of superior health. Our social life took bloom and it was nice to be with people again. We even joined the Detroit chapter of the American Natural Hygiene Society and attended meetings so we could further our knowledge, and, in addition, support this worthy organization. I became active in sports again: tennis, swimming, ice skating, and particularly my greatest love, baseball.

I looked back and assessed the past year. It was not an easy one. I was not "cured." At least not the way I would like to be. There were many ruts along the road to recovery, but I could see enough improvement to know that subsequent fasts and an adherence to this new way of life would be stepping stones that would put me on higher levels of health each year. I tried not to become discouraged or depressed, but it was difficult because I had been so sick for so long that the slightest deviation from what I considered normal at this point threw me into deep depressions. I guess it could be called a conditioned response from past years. It was tough to learn patience, but this is one virtue which pays dividends after it is learned.

This first year passed so quickly it just didn't seem possible the date was fast approaching for me to leave my home, family, and practice again for another fast. As much as I subconsciously rationalized about prolonging my departure, deep down I knew I had to go and wanted to go. I settled whatever business necessary and my good friend Newt (Dr. Karp) agreed to work my office again two days a week, which was one big load off my mind because there had to be an income source for my family.

I left for Hyde Park, New York, on August 4, 1965. It was the same time and the same train, but no sadness this time, only anticipation of great things to come. I didn't even bring along the "last supper" as I did last year. The trip was uneventful and I arrived at Pawling Manor more alive than last year, checked in, and began what was to be a four-week fast under the supervision of Dr. Gross.

Since I had been fasting one or two days a week the past year, the internal environment of my body was fairly clean. So, as much work as fasting is, this was an easier fast because of my being "cleaner." However, this fast, as well as future fasts, were very "productive." In other words, my body got right into it, my weight loss was more rapid, elimination of the toxic load began almost immediately, my tongue became heavily coated, breath and taste extremely foul much sooner, and my blood pressure lowered more rapidly. Actually, as one takes these long fasts and lives "hygienically" in between, then only shorter fasts are needed to accomplish what the earlier longer fasts did. (Now, 12 years later, I can take a one-, two-, or three-week fast and it would be about the equivalent of double its length.)

In the first six days of this fast, I lost 14 pounds; then it tapered down and only small amounts of weight were lost each day. There was varied bowel activity during the

first two weeks of the fast, ranging from one to four occurrences a day, but nowhere near the problem it was
last year. During the last two weeks, there were almost
no B.M.s except for an occasional spasm or two. There
were a few times I felt so low that Dr. Gross gave me a
few sips of diluted orange juice to bring my blood sugar
level up a bit and then I was able to go on.

Similar changes took place as in my first fast last
year: visual acuity increased; hearing, smell, and other
senses sharpened; increase in mental clarity; but above
all a great feeling of well-being and an inner strength. I
knew that more healing had taken place. I could feel it,
yet I didn't want to become overconfident lest I lose
everything I had fought so hard to attain; but there was
no chance of that now.

At the end of four weeks, Dr. Gross broke my fast as
carefully as last year, with the exception that, since I
had been conditioned to a basically raw vegetarian diet,
the raw, whole vegetables, fruits, and nuts were instituted
much earlier after the first few critical days of breaking
the fast. (There is always a thrill and nervous excitement
when breaking a fast, no matter how often one fasts. I
experienced these sensations on every fast.) The food,
simple as it is, has the most indescribable, fantastic, unbelievable taste immediately following a fast.

I spent two weeks more at Pawling, until the end of
September, 1965, building strength and weight, while
Dr. Gross observed how I was handling my vegetarian
diet. When he was satisfied that I was ready to return
home and blend back into my practice and home life,
he discharged me from his care and gave me advice—as
a father might give a son—on how to live in the ensuing
years, physically, mentally, and emotionally.

Corinne was waiting in the depot for me as my train arrived. It was different from last year. There was no fanfare, no heavy emotion or crying. We just embraced and went home. This was part of our way of life now for a while and we accepted these absences from each other because we both knew the ultimate goal.

Irwin and Darryl were so happy to see me. Even our two cats, who were participating part time in the vegetarian diet, demonstrated an outward show of affection. We spent hours talking about this latest experience, the things I saw and did, the recipes from Pawling, and the many people I met with so many health problems who were helped. This made me recall the many times I tried to thank Dr. Gross for helping me and he would always say, "I didn't do a thing but supervise your fast. You did it all yourself."

There was a little more improvement after this fast, which did much for my psyche. Again, I wasn't "cured" at this point but the handwriting was on the wall. I knew I could only go in one direction and that was forward. I had my ups and downs in this year and my discouraging moments, but they were to become fewer and fewer. The B.M.s were more or less formed now and their frequency would vary from two to six times a day. This was a far cry from the days of my medical treatment, and I have not taken any drugs thus far and I feel wonderful. Oh, there were still times when the "urge" came on strong and little accidents occurred, but they also became fewer.

Over the next three years (1966, 1967, and 1968), I undertook successive fasts of five-, four-, and five-weeks' duration. The 1966 and 1967 fasts were taken at Pawling, while the 1968 fast was undertaken at my home and supervised by me, although I did call Dr. Gross once a week to report my progress and receive guidance if needed. Each of these three fasts put me on higher plateaus of health, until I would estimate I was functioning about 75 to 80 percent of normal.

The five-week fast I took at home was not the best experience. I not only don't recommend a long fast at home, but I would discourage anyone from trying it only because the environment is not conducive to a proper fast. There are too many disturbing and enervating influences that actually detract from the beneficial effects: well-meaning friends and relatives intimating you're a little crazy; neighborhood noise from loud cars, motorcycles, and children; the smell of pollution from the city, from auto exhausts, and from people walking by the house smoking; plus a hundred and one other disturbances. You see, during a fast you become very sensitive to everything and are annoyed by the slightest irritation which ordinarily might not bother you if you were not fasting. This upsets the entire system and can cause the fast to be detrimental. The ideal and safest way is to have the long fasts supervised by professionals at a hygienic institution.

From 1969 to the present (1976), I fasted one or two days a week. Several times a year I'll put together a three- or four-day fast. The vegetarian diet (with the foods properly combined, as will be explained later) has been strictly adhered to over these years and meat has literally become repugnant to me. Through the proper use of all the principles of Natural Hygiene, I feel I have just about reached the top of the plateau, though I continue to notice minute changes in the improvement of my general physical, mental, and emotional health. I would say to date, 1976, I am functioning about 95 percent or more of normal and one day I may even surpass that. The 5 percent or less is due to damage (adhesions) in the colon from the prolonged debility which occurred during the six years under medical care. I feel I'm damn lucky to have been able to recuperate to this point and it's quite possible these adhesions can be reduced even further because the magnificent power of the human body cannot be underestimated. The body is self-constructing, self-defending, self-repairing, and self-regulating. It is so sad when people use Natural Hygiene as an eleventh hour measure, as I did, but are beyond their recuperative capabilities and cannot save their organs or their lives. Natural Hygiene is lived, not so much for the recuperation from illness, but for its most important asset—the evolution of vigorous health and the prevention of disease.

I've watched my wife blossom into a new woman, her natural beauty being enhanced by a youthful look that surprises people who assume she is thirtyish and then discover she is past 42. It is the sum total of all our experiences over these past years—1958 to 1976—from the inception of my illness until the present that has made us totally committed to Natural Hygiene and to its perpetuation.

Corinne and I eventually became officers in the Detroit chapter of the American Natural Hygiene Society and have built it into the largest, most active chapter in the country. We then became involved in the national organization—The American Natural Hygiene Society—and eventually were elected to the board of directors. I currently have the honor of being the president and official representative of the American Natural Hygiene Society.

I willingly give up time from my practice, sometimes

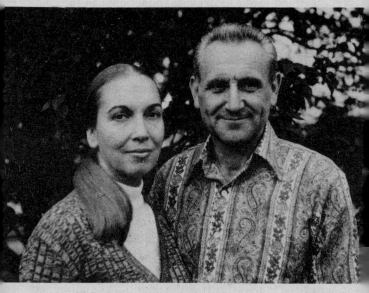

Dr. Jack Goldstein and his wife, Corinne.

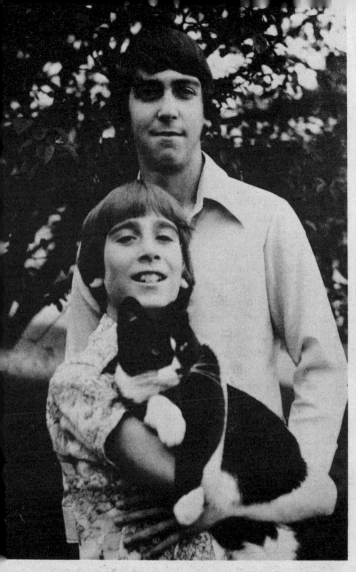

Dr. Goldstein's two sons, Irwin, 16 years old, and Darryl, 13 years old, both raised as vegetarians for the last 12 years. Also pictured is the boys' pet cat, Pokey.

more time than I can afford, to lecture and do radio and television shows all over the United States and Canada. This has allowed me to come in contact with, and have a profound influence on, many thousands of people and their lives. I think this has been the most gratifying experience for me, to be able to play a part in altering and bettering peoples' lives.

Life with Natural Hygiene has afforded me countless unusual experiences, some humorous and some pathetic, of which I'd like to share just a few. There was the time I was making plans to move into a new office building and I dropped in on the workmen one morning to go over some of my electrical and plumbing needs, etc. I was offered coffee and doughnuts, which I refused, and one thing led to another and before I knew it there was a discussion of why I refused these morning goodies, the virtues of natural living, and the vegetarian diet. The men seemed fascinated by the discussion and obviously one of them had never come in contact with a vegetarian before, because when I was preparing to leave, one of the men approached me, shook my hand and said, "I've enjoyed listening to you and it was a pleasure to meet you because I've never met a 'vegetable man' before."

It seems most people are of the opinion that ill health is the normal sequence in the pattern of their lives. They have come to accept disease, if they live long enough, as the norm because "most everyone gets sick." It is good health that is normal to the body. I run across many examples, in my office, of people who have these warped opinions of health and disease. But I'll always remember this patient from whom I was obtaining a history. This is a classic. In questioning her about her medical history, she said, as she lit up a cigarette, "I have arthritis, high blood pressure, psoriasis, asthma and emphysema, but other than that, I'm in good health." Need I say more?

This incident occurred at the University of Windsor, Windsor, Ontario, Canada (1974). It was the American Natural Hygiene Society's annual conference on natural living. I had just delivered a lecture entitled "My Six-Week Fast," which was the basic story in this book. A gentleman approached me, shook my hand, complimented me on my lecture, and introduced himself as Dr.———— (I cannot use his name), a medical doctor from Kansas. (There are many medical doctors as well as other medical practitioners who attend our conferences.) He said he had attended other conferences of the A.N.H.S. and this was the third time he had heard my lecture and he just wanted to tell me that "your story is a classic example of the abuses the human body is subjected to by the medical profession."

A rather disgusting situation arose recently when I entered a branch office of the Michigan Cancer Foundation to pick up a projector, a movie film, and literature pertaining to smoking and lung cancer. Once inside, I did everything but choke from the heavy curtain of cigarette smoke that hung like a thick fog. I observed four women workers. Three of them were smoking and there were four packs of cigarettes on the table, assuring them they wouldn't run short before the day was over. One of the women gave me the projector, the smoking and cancer film, and a stack of anti-smoking literature, while a burning cigarette dangled from her lips. They laughed when I questioned the stupidity of what they were doing, but I couldn't pursue it any further because by this time my eyes and lungs were burning and I had to get out of there. I did report the incident to the Michigan Cancer Foundation and was told this does happen, but they would look into it. So guess what? Right! They're still smoking and passing out information on lung cancer.

Of all the many other experiences I could continue with, this final example is probably the most relevant and had the most profound impact on Corinne and me. It started with a newspaper article I saw in the Detroit News in 1972 concerning the National Foundation for Ileitis and Colitis. The ideals, purpose, and goals were presented. The address of the president was given, which was in New York. I located his telephone number, called him, and explained my interest in helping people and what my new simple way of life held as a potential, not only for helping those afflicted, but as a means of preventing these problems. He stated he couldn't do much and that I should contact a certain medical doctor at the University of Colorado Medical Center in Denver, which I did by phone. I was instructed to write a letter, which I also did, requesting to speak at a conference he was chairing. He wrote back and said it was impossible for me to participate in the conference and casually mentioned how interesting my case seemed and that he would pass along this information to his colleagues "because such information is of value in enhancing our knowledge." Needless to say, the information was not passed along and needless to say that this attitude is what I continually run up against when I confront medical men with this simple, logical, and physiologically sound alternative to their current and frustrating methods of treatment. You would think that since the welfare of the hu-

man being is the *only* purpose for the existence of doctors
that they would leave no doors unopened if there was
any way possible that their fellow man (or woman)
could be helped. But they won't listen. It seems the biggest concern of the Foundation is to collect money for
research and cures. Cures? No cure can ever better the
body's own innate capability to heal itself.

It was this knowledge of the Foundation that made
Corinne and me aware of a meeting to be held at a major
hospital for the purpose of organizing a Detroit chapter
of the National Foundation for Ileitis and Colitis. We
attended that meeting in May of 1975. There were
hundreds of sick people packed into the auditorium. Some
were in early stages of "treatment," some had been under
"treatment" for many years, while others had already been
subjected to that drastic surgery. There were young children, elderly people, and all the ages in between. They
were all sick and they were all there to learn about the
advances (?) made in the treatment of digestive diseases.
A faint cloud of smoke floated lazily in the room because
at least one-fourth of the people were smoking.

The distinguished panel of five doctors was introduced.
Dr. Kale was among this group. Each spoke of his experiences and discussed the rationale of various "treatments." The use of the high-protein diet was advocated
to build up the patient. However, many of these patients
did not have the capacity to properly absorb and assimilate food (convert the nutriment into living tissue), especially a high-protein diet which puts an extra tax on
the kidneys, liver, and body in general since it requires
much more energy for its digestion. And one thing the
sick body does not have is energy. What energy it does

have should be conserved and directed toward recuperation. Why is a broken arm put in a cast? So it may rest and thereby heal. How then can a diseased intestine, particularly in ulcerative colitis, be expected to heal when all this food is being forced into it? The intestine is never given a chance to rest.

Another item brought up by one of the panel was, "We have to wait for better drugs to come along." What are these drugs supposed to do? How is disease to be cured by any drug? I have yet to have a question answered that I have been asking for years: "How does a drug cure?" The panelist did concede that "any drug we ever give has risks to it." It can be stated that all drugs are dangerous.

Surgery was also discussed. This is drastic and traumatic, as I've already mentioned. The surgeon stated, "There is a high recurrence rate after surgical treatment. Many times, multiple surgery in a patient follows." The Foundation states that there are about 25 to 45 percent recurrences following surgery. They also state that "for all practical purposes, ulcerative colitis can be cured by removing the entire colon and establishing an ileostomy. Even this removal of the colon and establishing an ileostomy does not invariably prevent spread of the disease to higher segments of the bowel." For all practical purposes, headaches can be cured by cutting off the head, however, this *does* cure the headache. The excision of the entire colon removes only the end result of a pathological process—it does not remove cause. This can apply to disease in general. Unless cause is removed, the disease cannot be considered as "cured." By the same token, when a disease is suppressed, as with drugs, the cause has not been eliminated and therefore the body may break out in another disease eventually.

Dr. Kale, in his presentation, stated that, "The disease can be removed surgically." Can it? He also stated that, "Diet has nothing to do with the history of the disease in any way." One cannot isolate the colon from any other part of the body, just as one cannot isolate any part from the whole. The body functions as a unit and when one part suffers or malfunctions or becomes diseased, then the whole body is affected. The improper and debilitated foods people eat today can hardly allow them to evolve good general health. This is one of the keys. Just as one improves on a fast, feels marvelous when it's over, and puts in his body "live" foods that will allow the evolution of a high degree of health, so this person will find if he returns to his "normal" way of eating (if he wants to live that dangerously) that eventually he will have lost all he had gained and is back in the same rut as before.

When the discussions ended, questions were taken from the audience on 3 × 5 cards and given to the panel. While the cards were being collected, I turned to Corinne and we both agreed that in the 18 years since I first became ill, nothing had changed. Time had stood still. The same principles of treatment, the same search for cures and new drugs, and the same closed minds, amazingly, but not surprisingly, still existed. The many cards were screened by the panel and then they began reading and answering the questions. We had sent in a question concerning fasting, which was selected by Dr. Kale. He so completely misled and misinformed the audience, especially since his experience with fasting could probably be put on the head of a pin, that Corinne could not take any more of it. She stood up and wanted to be heard, even though no oral questions were being taken. She told the panel and the audience that the answer was misleading and too quickly pushed aside. She wanted the panel and the audience to at least listen to what we had to say about our experience (which is also the experience of untold thousands of others), to at least become aware that there is a way to be helped. She was immediately put down by the moderator, which angered her even more. Corinne then strongly accused him of suppressing information from these people, many of whom were desperate. He still put her down, but she was adamant and again accused him of suppression. There began a scattered applause from the audience with a few voices ringing out such things as, "Let them speak," "Let's hear what they have to say," etc. The moderator was finally pressured into inviting us up to the front of the auditorium; but our little victory was to be short-lived. As we approached the front, I could see the panel quickly huddling for the final blow. They were not to be outdone. Before we could open our mouths, the moderator emphatically called the meeting to an end and summoned help from the security guard. Amazing! Corinne and I created all that fear and danger by ourselves.

What followed next, I had seen in newsreels and newspapers but never imagined it would happen to us. The security guard arrived (without bugles and fanfare) and grabbed, quite firmly, those two dangerous people (us). For lack of a more dignified description, the guard "threw us out," much to the dissatisfaction of the many people who followed us outside to seek more information.

It wasn't ten minutes later that the security guard returned and invited us back in at the request of one of the doctors (who probably thought we were harmless—but we carry a strong message). The doctor briefly and superficially discussed fasting with me. I later asked him if he was interested in the evolvement of good general health in his patients, rather than just the condition of their intestines. He said he was; so I asked why such a large number of the sick people here tonight, most of whom were patients of his and of the other members of the panel, were permitted to smoke. He pondered a moment and then hesitatingly said it was a good point. How unaware can one be?

Then, as Corinne and I were getting ready to leave, Dr. Kale walked by and we shook hands. He told me that this fasting and the entire plan of natural living was a "religion." What do you say to one who has studied the human body, yet has so little awareness of its needs?

It is the culmination of many such confrontations that has taught me to mistake not authority for truth, but rather to make truth my authority.

It is this latter type of experience that not only disappoints me, but keeps me continually frustrated because, generally speaking, doctors don't want to listen—at least not with an open mind. But I'll tell you who *will* listen, and this is where the education should be directed: to the people—the everyday person like you or your neighbor. After all, that's what it's all about—helping people!

This brings the story of a very personal part of my life to a conclusion, although in reality it is merely a continuation of the beginning, since my life goes on from here. I am thankful I *have* life; but I am even more thankful that I can share this life of bountiful and unequivocal "good health."

PART II

CHAPTER VIII

The Magnificent Power of the Body—Case Histories I've Observed

Over the past 12 years, I've had the opportunity to witness countless cases of recovery from disease, in my repeated sojourns to Pawling Manor and in my travels in the United States and Canada. The healing power of the body is so remarkable that if I had not actually seen some of these recoveries, I probably would not have believed it. I could write a book on case histories, but there are some being written now and I only want to present a few cases that stand out in my mind as most dramatic so you can appreciate the body's tremendous potential and ability to achieve normalcy.

My first roommate at Pawling Manor in 1964 was a gentleman (let's call him L. P.) of 68 years of age. He had come there a chronically ill man who had been through the usual medical treatments. He was obese, had an enlarged prostate, and Bright's disease (a kidney disease in which there is high blood pressure plus albumin in the urine). He fasted 52 days (just drank water), during which time his weight came down, his blood pressure lowered, his prostate problem cleared, and he was able to urinate normally and without albumin. He felt marvelous and looked younger than his age at the termination of the fast. I remember near the termination of his fast that he began throwing up bile. It was black bile. This was a crisis (as I explained back in the ninth day of my fast) that sometimes occurs during a fast and it was allowing the body to eliminate some of its deep-seated "junk" of many years accumulation. When the vomiting phase passed, there was marked improvement. To show me how much weight he lost, L. P. put his entire body into one pant leg of his trousers. After a number of weeks on the vegetarian diet, L. P. went home a happy man.

Shortly after L. P. went home, I acquired another roommate. He was a young man who was virtually blind in one eye and was partially blind but rapidly losing the sight in the other eye. Doctors didn't know why this was happening or how to stop it, so J. G. had nothing to lose by trying a fast. He fasted three weeks and was put on a completely raw vegetarian diet. The blind eye did not respond, but the other eye improved just enough so he could read, which he could not do previously. His body was only able to repair that which was not irreversible, which wasn't too much, but at least there was some improvement and J. G. left there with a way of life that would allow him to improve his general health and that of his family.

There's an elderly man I've met several times at Pawling. He is in fine health and has no problems, but he comes up every year for several weeks. He fasts one week and eats a strict vegetarian diet the next week. This is

M. F.'s insurance premium he pays to stay in good health. It recharges his battery, so to speak.

J. D. is a young man I met my first and second year at the Manor. The first time he was there because of a nephritis (kidney disease) and kidney stones. He refused medical treatment because surgery was recommended and he did not want to be cut open and all that goes with it. He fasted about 40 days and during the last few days he was urinating into filter paper. His body had broken down the stones and they were passing as gravel into the filter paper and they could be seen. The nephritis cleared and after three weeks on a strict vegetarian diet of mostly raw fruits, vegetables, and nuts, he went home. I saw him again the following year. He said he had no more problems with the kidney, but now he had some large varicose veins and a large clot at the inner side of the knee where the great saphenous vein makes its turn. You see, J. D. was a carpenter who squatted most of the day and the constant pressure caused the vein problem. He fasted three weeks, during which time I watched and palpated the veins and clot. The varicose veins gradually returned to normal and the clot disappeared; however, we must remember two things. First is that if J. D. returns to squatting again, then the same causative factors are operating again, and second, he responded well because the valves in the veins were competent. If the valves were incompetent and of no use, then the results would not have been good.

J. D.'s wife had a most dramatic experience several years previously. She was diagnosed as having a fibroid tumor of the uterus and was advised to have a hysterectomy. She refused surgery because she wanted to keep her organs intact, if possible. Her fast was about 30 days' duration. She later returned to her gynecologist, who, after a pelvic examination, saw no evidence of the fibroid tumor and was frankly amazed.

Another of my roommates was a man who was seventyish, had high blood pressure, and was obese. J. S. also had arthritis (generalized) and a locked hip joint. His pain was almost constant, particularly in the joints of his hands, and he had lived for years on large daily doses of Bufferin. J. S. had been fasting four or five days when one morning I was startled out of a sound sleep by his yelling. After the cobwebs cleared from my head, I asked what was wrong and he said he was fine. It was just that he was so elated because this was the first time in years that he had not taken Bufferin for so long and not had pain. In fact, he quickly flexed and extended his wrists and fingers to demonstrate the freedom of motion, which had not been present for a long time. J. S. fasted four weeks and followed a very careful, basically raw, vegetarian diet. His weight and blood pressure came down, his generalized joint pain subsided and his joints were able to function more freely. His locked hip joint remained locked, but he had just a little more motion in it, which made it easier for him to ambulate. His hip was also free of pain. The reason it remained locked is that there is a certain amount of irreversibility. Once a joint has eroded, there's not much chance for a return to normal.

I've seen people who wanted to give up smoking, but all attempts failed. After about a ten day to two week fast, the habit was broken. When they tried to smoke, they became nauseated and ill. Some became violently sick. Through the fast, their bodies had become clean and it didn't take much internal pollution to cause these reactions. There is one important fact: You must sincerely and without a doubt want to quit smoking.

The fast, followed by a natural hygienic way of living, will give the body the best chance for survival. This applies to everyone who says goodbye to their former living habits, particularly the "fatties"—the obese. They probably have more chronic illness, more debilitating and degenerative diseases, more liver, kidney, diabetic, stroke and heart problems, etc., than anyone else. This does not preclude a shorter life span. The obese probably benefit more than anyone from the Natural Hygiene way of life. The weight will stay down, the blood pressure will stay down, the organs are given a chance to improve, and general health will markedly improve, giving the body the only real and sound chance for an increased life span free of disease.

Mrs. E. B. suffered for years with ileitis (similar to colitis but involving the lower end of the small intestine). It was quite debilitating and made life quite miserable since it necessitated her always being near a lavatory. She was weak, generally run-down, and didn't have that "spark." She spent most of her time at home. Eventually, part of the small intestine closed off (obstruction), which was not only extremely painful but a threat to life. Surgery was performed on E. B., consisting of the cutting out of one and one-half feet of intestine and joining the cut ends with the same length of plastic tubing. Actually, the problem was not corrected because only the end result of a pathological process was removed. Cause was not removed, nor were any requisites of life supplied. So is it any wonder that several years later another obstruction occurred and surgical removal of another section of intestine was advised. By this time E. B. was aware of Natural Hygiene and decided to get involved. She went to a hygienic institution and fasted for four weeks. During the fast, improvement was evident. The discomfort and the obstruction disappeared. She was guided very carefully onto a vegetarian diet. Subsequent long and short fasts have been taken each year, elevating her to higher levels of health to the point where she enjoys life again and looks forward to going out and socializing. She is eating foods her doctors said she could not handle, but are the doctors interested in her case? Are they curious about her progress? No! The severe diarrhea eventually eased and bowel action improved toward normalcy, although because of severe damage in the intestine from years of abuse under medical care and because of the length of plastic tubing that substitutes for part of the intestine, there are periodic ups and downs. But these little annoyances are trivial compared to the new lease on life achieved.

I've seen cases of so-called allergy disappear after a fast and in many cases after only a change in diet with the observance of proper combining of foods (which will be explained and clarified later). People who were supposed to be allergic to tomatoes or strawberries, pollen, wool, dust, animal danders, etc., have become free of these so-called sensitivities, which means merely that their bodies are functioning at an optimum level of health. I recall two women. One was "allergic" to tomatoes and the other was allergic to rabbit fur. Now I doubt if this will make world-shattering history, but after fasting and being put on the proper diet of natural foods, the one woman ate several tomatoes with no ill effects and the other woman had a hat made of rabbit fur and suffered no ill effects.

Asthma is another problem which responds almost dramatically to a fast and to a vegetarian diet. Many asthmatics experience crises during the fast, such as varying degrees of asthmatic attacks, but when they understand that they are temporary they are not as frightened as they might have been. These crises readily pass and then the individual finds it difficult to believe the new freedom with which he can breathe. Once the body eliminates its internal toxic load and becomes clean via the fast, then it's all downhill. Some people, for one reason or another, can't or don't want to fast and they watch their diet, food combinations, emotions, etc. They also obtain a nice response, but it is usually slower than if they had fasted. Of course, there are many other factors in allergy and asthma, not the least of which are the intake of such things as coffee, chocolate, white flour and white sugar products, denatured-processed-preserved-and-embalmed foods, meat, milk, drugs and medicines, wheat, eggs, food additives . . . the list is an endless array of most of the constitutents of conventional or "normal" living.

I have seen cases of diabetes and its antithesis, hypoglycemia (low blood sugar), both benefit from a properly supervised fast. In some of the cases of diabetes, the people were actually able to give up insulin. In other cases, the insulin was able to be minimized. The big factor in the improvement of health was the changeover from the refined, denatured, and chemicalized diet to the natural diet. Generally speaking, when all the needs of life are supplied, good health is the ultimate result, unless the body has deteriorated so far as to be beyond its own capacity to recover.

Mrs. R. C., 25 years of age, developed ileitis. There was diarrhea, intestinal spasm, bleeding, abdominal cramps, and gradual debility. For three years she underwent the usual medical treatment of tranquilizers, antibiotics, antispasmodics (smooth muscle relaxants to reduce intestinal motility), a mushy diet devoid of much nourishment, and a variety of pain killer drugs. She eventually reached a point of extreme pain accompanied by fever which her doctor diagnosed as an obstruction. There was no response to treatment except that the problem worsened. The doctor advised cutting out about one and a half feet of intestine. R. C. was aware of Natural Hygiene, but had no desire to utilize this knowledge until now; she did not want to subject herself to surgery. She was made to realize, by me (she is my sister), that the surgery would not eliminate the cause of her problems and that her pattern of living would remain unchanged. She would not be taught how to live properly, how to evolve good health, or how to prevent an inevitable recurrence of the problem. So she decided to become involved in Natural Hygiene, since she had nothing to lose. She could always have the operation if this method didn't allow her to help herself, but once the section of intestine is cut out, it is gone forever. So this seemed logical to her, particularly since she saw the fantastic progress of my own case. She went away to a hygienic institution where she fasted a total of five weeks. It was during the first week of the fast that the extreme pain (which was so intense she could not lie on her abdomen) subsided, the obstruction released, and she was able to sleep on her tummy without discomfort. Her weight, which was much in excess, came down. She almost could not believe how marvelous she looked and felt after the fast was terminated and she began eating vegetarian fare. R. C. was so elated, she carried home this enthusiasm and began the conversion of her two little girls (and eventually her husband) to the natural way of life so they too could enjoy a life free of disease. R. C. required subsequent fasts and a close adherence to the Natural Hygiene principles, but the return of her health was the eventual outcome—a health far exceeding her expectations. As of this writing (1976), she is 31 years old and enjoys premium health.

I've observed dramatic results from both fasting and/or a basically raw vegetarian diet in the treatment of psoriasis, so-called eczemas, and other skin problems. Of course, many skin problems are nothing more than the body's own eliminative mechanism in action. In fact, many times on a fast the skin may erupt temporarily with an acne-type condition. This is one of the many channels through which the body can rid itself of its accumulated toxic (poisonous) wastes. I recall, deep in my first fast, the development of a facial acne which gradually cleared as the internal environment of my body became cleaner. There are so many exotic medicines, ointments, creams, and lotions (none of which gets at causes) with which to treat the myriad dermatitis problems that it borders on the ridiculous to see them resolve with the judicious use of the fast and avoidance of the "conventional" diet and other poisonous habits already mentioned elsewhere in this book.

J. F. suffered a massive heart attack about six months

before coming to Pawling Manor. He had a myocardial infarction (death of an area of heart muscle), an aortic aneurysm (thinning and weakening with a slight ballooning out of a part of the wall of the main artery coming out of the heart; there is an ever-present danger of this area rupturing, with internal bleeding leading to death very quickly), and was overweight with high blood pressure. His doctors advised him to give up his work, to stay as much as possible in his third-floor apartment, which had no elevator, and to take various "heart" medicines. He began living the life of a hermit and in constant fear. Someone told him of a better way—Natural Hygiene—and sketchily familiarized him with it. J. F. decided to give it a try and went to the Manor in the fall of 1964, my first time there also. I was in the fourth week of my fast when he arrived. He really did not know what to expect and had built up a fear. It was for this reason he was not put on a fast right away, but on a strictly raw vegetarian diet—just fruits, vegetables, and small amounts of nuts for about ten days to two weeks, until he learned more of what he was to experience and had overcome his unfounded but understandable fear. It was during this time Dr. Gross advised J. F. to pay me a visit to see a person in the fourth week of a fast so some confidence could be developed. J. F. was surprised to see me looking and feeling as well as I did. He asked me many questions concerning my fast and I reassured him. When I first saw J. F. he had a gray, ashen complexion. I've seen this type of complexion in many heart cases. The simple act of getting out of a chair and walking across the room caused fatigue and labored breathing. During this feeding cycle I watched him improve to the degree that his complexion became normal, his weight and blood pressure dropped markedly, and he was able to take walks without the fatigue and strain previously encountered. J. F. was then put on a fast which turned out to be of four weeks' duration. At its termination he was fed very strictly on a raw vegetarian diet for about two weeks and then put on another fast for two weeks. He did not take any medication during his entire stay or after leaving. Some time later he returned to his cardiologist for an examination. The doctor was in a state of disbelief when he found no evidence of the infarct (as explained previously) and no evidence of the aneurysm, even on x-ray study. J. F.'s weight and blood pressure was maintained within normal limits. All of this happened without the use of drugs. J. F. returned to his job, which required him to travel extensively. He also conquered the stairs at his third-floor apartment. But the important point is that instead of vegetating as he was instructed by his doctors, and living in constant fear, he was now able to grab a chunk of precious life and hold onto it.

Recently I received a long distance telephone call from a Mrs. M.D. concerning her husband who was hospitalized with colitis. The doctors did not know quite what to do at this point and Mrs. D. was extremely worried and frightened. I couldn't tell her what to do. I could only tell her about my case, what had happened and what fasting and the natural way of life had to offer. The decision had to be made by her and her husband. No one else could make it for them. A number of weeks lapsed and then I received correspondence from Mrs. D. from which I'd like to quote portions: "Well, D——— was transfered from B——— hospital to a Natural Hygiene retreat. Needless to say, I can't express in words how much your information and guidance helped me in making the decision to strongly influence my husband with regard to a change. I sincerely felt, call it an inner feeling, that had D——— remained in the hospital, he would have died—or perhaps even worse had a colostomy or colectomy or such. In my heart, I felt D——— should have gone to a hygienic institution at the beginning. I should have followed that feeling. It was a correct one. The doctor told me I was psychotic. D———'s family was against me and I was afraid to do anything for fear that what I'd decide might be wrong. But one thing I forgot to trust in—and that is my love for D———. After talking to you, Dr. Goldstein, I felt you had reinforced my first thoughts and what I wanted to do was the only logical and sensible thing to do. Thank you for helping me to help my husband."

Another letter came two months later and in part went: "We are so pleased with D———'s results. He has no colostomy, no drug poisoning with its many 'sicknesses' and no multiple bowel movements. I feel that you were able to help us arrive at a sensible and very pleasant end result through fasting."

These are not just isolated letters that I receive. These are only a few of the many dozens received from people all over the country and from all walks of life who allowed the seeds of knowledge I planted in their minds to sprout, take root and grow. It is not my purpose here to print an endless assortment of letters, but rather to give you an idea of how people are thinking. Of course there are cases that don't, or can't, recover because the damage has gone beyond the body's ability to recuperate, but in many cases of terminal illness such as intractable lung cancer, fasting has permitted the unfortunate individual to die in peace without becoming a narcotics addict.

While undertaking my third fast at the Manor (this one of five weeks' duration) in 1966, I met a most remarkable woman. We arrived and began our fasts on the same day, but we didn't meet until several days later. She had multiple sclerosis and had run the gamut of medical treatments. When her doctors finally gave up on her, M. R. could only walk about ten minutes and then had to lie down due to weakness. Although her doctors gave up, she did not. She knew there must be a way to beat this terrible affliction. M. R. discovered Natural Hygiene and made a decision to go away to fast and alter her entire way of life. It was a difficult fast for her, but she and I broke our fasts on the same day five weeks later. M——— spent most of the time in bed resting, but she would occasionally sit out in the sun for short periods. After a carefully broken fast and two weeks on a strictly raw vegetarian diet, she was able to walk for 20 minutes— that's double what she was able to do previously. I kept in touch with M——— after leaving the Manor and followed her remarkable progress. Soon she could put in a half day of work, though she was quite tired. Her endurance increased as time went on—and so did her level of health. She was taking no drugs. I received a Christmas card from M——— in 1968, two years after her first fast and her adoption of the vegetarian diet and hygienic way of living. I'll try to break down her letter to me, since M——— was from Canada but bilingual (on the French side). She said she had taken subsequent fasts since 1966. "I really think I will get rid of this M. S. sickness. I went to Montreal Expo '67 every night, came back at 12 at night, and worked the next day. Never tired; always in good shape. I feel like 15. Jack, I tell you it is so good to be alive. I'll never again be unhappy. Nothing upsets me. I have to stop and think that I am an M. S. case. Though I can't but little run yet, I jumped 20 to 25 times in the air with a rope. The doctors say I have a remission and it will start again but I laugh at that. It is all they can say. I tell them how is it I have my remission when I want to? I educate others, for I know many M. S. cases." I received another Christmas card in 1969. To quote in part, M———— says, "As far as my health is concerned, I'm almost cured, though the hardship of life doesn't help. But I am almost cured after four fasts and an adequate hygienic way of living. It's wonderful to be alive again.

"I have more energy. Never, never tired. I feel great, wonderful. I'm always happy and nothing will darken my future. I found everything when I found the way to walk again. I walk and walk for hours. I feel I am eternal and I'll never be sick again." What else can I add at this point? Anything said now would just be anticlimax.

CHAPTER IX

A Glance at Fad Diets and Food Additives

Since we are interested in total health, particularly prevention of disease and not just the health of a part of the body, it behooves us to be aware of other factors that could be detrimental to good health. This chapter will not deal in great depth with fad diets or food additives, but will give you a smattering of information to enlighten you and increase your awareness. *You* make your own decisions.

Gluttony is probably the worst dietetic sin. Most people suffer from overeating—eating beyond their digestive capacities. They also suffer from the harmful effects of haphazardly dumping in their stomachs an amazing variety of foods and half-foods in abominable combinations that would wreak havoc in the strongest of digestive systems. I'll cover the advantages and rationale of proper food combining in the next chapter.

Prevention magazine, July, 1973, states that "one of the worst things about low cholesterol diets is that they prohibit you almost entirely from eating liver, eggs, milk, cheese, beef, and shellfish, all of which are superlatively nutritious foods. Eliminate these foods from your diet and it is all but impossible to consume the vitamins, minerals and trace elements you need to keep your whole body in good health." This is a typical example of the common misconception most people have that without these foods one cannot live in good health. The fact is that it is the very people who eat these foods who flood the hospitals and doctors' offices with their anemias, arthritis, diabetes, kidney diseases, cancers, so-called allergies, colitis, and an endless list of degenerative diseases. It is not the scope of this chapter to analyze foods in depth, but cheese (if natural, unprocessed, unchemicalized, and unsalted) is probably the most innocuous of the bunch. The others have long-term harmful effects to the body. The ideal source of protein, vitamins, minerals, and trace elements comes from the plant kingdom—vegetables, fruits, nuts, seeds, and sprouts in their natural unfired (raw) state where possible—in which the inorganic elements of the soil are converted into living organic material, making all these elements biologically charged. If one is going to eat meat, then the only proper way to obtain all the nutrition is to eat the animal the way a carnivore would eat it—fresh-killed, uncooked, and including blood, bones, organs, and innards. If one cannot eat it this way, he shouldn't eat it at all. After all, where did that hunk of beef come from that is so "rich in protein and blood building elements"? It came from the steer that grazed and ate vegetation— the "greens." The meat-eaters thus get their protein second-hand in the food chain.

The Low Carbohydrate Diet seems to be an imbalanced diet with an overemphasis on protein. Today, people are over-proteinized and this can put a burden on the liver and kidneys.

The Nibbler's Diet—This is for people who think they must be eating all day. (Probably helps neurotics.)

Good Housekeeping Magazine Snacker's Diet—Similar to the Nibbler's Diet. To quote: "The key to this plan is six mini-meals a day so you may eat every few hours and never have time to be hungry." (Must cause problems, as the digestive system and body are never given a rest.) Recommended for the in-between snack meals are such things as jam, crackers, and ice cream which are "especially filling and nutritious." (What can I say about this junk.) Also allowed are pretzel sticks, shrimp in cocktail sauce, small cans of juice, and diet soda. Very little raw, fresh natural food is used. This has got to be a contributing factor in the propagation of disease.

It's In to Be Thin and *Dr. Cantor's Longevity Diet*—Basically same gimmicks as other diets.

Drinking Man's Diet—I think that if you're not an alcoholic before you start, you could have a chance at becoming one by the time you're done.

Eat More to Lose Weight Diet—Same song. Excess protein, etc.

Grape Cure—Foods don't cure!

Eat Your Way to Health—Usual theme. Use of supplements is highly recommended. I like my own idea for a title to this diet: "Digging Your Grave With Your Teeth."

Biochemic Method—The use of unlimited types of chemical compounds for each ailment or desired result. (Hardly supplies the requisites of life.)

Juice Fasting Diet—Tells of the healing power of

juices and what juices are used for specific conditions. Juices have no power to heal, treat, or cure; juices don't act on the body, the body acts on the juices. Technically this is not really fasting because juices are foods and must be handled by the digestive apparatus, but to a lesser degree of expended energy than solid foods.

How to Cut Your Food Budget in Half and Still Get Proper Nutrition—Same story. But the only way to get proper nutrition is to eat hygienically; that is, a variety of vegetarian fare: raw fresh fruits, vegetables, nuts, seeds, and sprouts eaten in proper combination. Of course, if you desire to cut your food budget 100 percent, then fast (but not indefinitely or you'll also cut your earthly existence 100 percent). Most people are in need of a fast to sharpen the power of their digestive systems, thereby allowing the body to properly digest and assimilate (absorb and utilize) these vital foods which in turn contributes to proper nutrition.

Weight Watchers—How much canned tuna fish can one eat? There are chemical additives in their brand of foods. Fresh fruits and vegetables are used, which is fine. One will lose weight, but there is not much chance of evolving robust health that will continue into later years.

Alpine Team Training Diet for Women—This is a good one for cholesterol freaks, because in addition to black tea or coffee, a few fruits and vegetables, the dieter must consume over 2 dozen eggs a week. Put *that* in your coronary arteries!

Boston Police Diet—This diet is against bananas, dates, cherries, grapes, plums, pears, apples, rice, potatoes, corn, beets, beans, peas, and carrots. I didn't check to see if this diet was against Boston baked beans.

Ice Cream Diet—Quote: "A fun diet that will startle your friends and associates." I'd like to add on to this: "Of course they'll also be startled when you get your first heart attack."

The Only Diet That Works—I thought perhaps someone had the right idea but it turns out to be composed of the same gimmicks presented in a different way.

Dr. Atkins' Diet Revolution—Another imbalanced diet that can be dangerous to your health. It's a low-carbohydrate high-fat and high-protein diet. This diet allows an unlimited consumption of saturated fat and is a cholesterol-rich diet.

The Wonder Diet—Lets you eat generously of all the foods you enjoy: bread, certain fruits and vegetables, meat, chicken, fish, jello, coffee, tea, milk, plus all the Scotch, bourbon, rye, gin, vodka, and brandy you desire. You can have a big roast beef sandwich as a snack or a milk shake as often as every hour of the day. This diet is stated to be "medically safe for patients with diabetes, high blood pressure, and heart conditions." Now, you might lose weight from this diet, but how you can develop anything but ill health, eventually, I can't imagine. I can't see how it can be safe for the above-mentioned diseases when one is allowed such generous amounts of poisons as coffee, tea, milk shakes every hour, beef, and booze. The only reason I can see for the name of this Wonder Diet is that it will be a wonder if you don't become very ill and/or succumb eventually.

Macrobiotics—This is primarily a grain and rice diet and is highly acid-forming. Nutritional balance is ignored. Fresh fruits and vegetables are not recommended or used unless in season, which means people in the north have them available only a few months out of the year. There is great importance placed on cooked food. It's cooking that devitalizes food and takes the life out of it.

Stillman Diet—Vitamin supplements are used. It's a low-residue diet, meaning less of the important roughage. This means fewer bowel movements and even sluggish bowel movements. This can predispose to intestinal and colon diseases. But the main ideas are the unlimited consumption of meat, eggs, sea food, etc., and the ingestion of at least eight glasses of water a day (whether your body needs it or not) in addition to the black coffee, tea, and diet soda (all poisons to the human body) you are encouraged to drink. Now, in the latest Stillman Protein-Plus diet, the liquid requirement has been increased to ten glasses of any combination of "permitted drinks." All this liquid causes frequent urination and can result in a mineral depletion from the constant flushing of the system. If there is any history of liver or kidney disease, a high-protein diet can be dangerous. If there is no history of liver or kidney diseases, then could it be quite possible to develop some on a prolonged high-protein diet?

Martinis and Whipped Cream—"Eat as much and as often as you want. Enjoy those two or three martinis before dinner and that brandy after dinner. Enjoy fried foods such as pork sausages, etc., gravies, dressings, ice cream, and whipped cream." This diet is set up so you can lose weight, but I don't see anything but ill health developing from it.

Brand Name Diet—This is probably the worst abomination of all. To quote: "A remarkable new diet based on frozen, packaged, and canned food available in every supermarket." Can you possibly imagine the dangerous cumulative effects from living off of a diet of foodless foods loaded with chemical food additives?

Psychologists' Eat-Anything Diet—"The foods you crave are the ones you should eat. Foods that merely 'beckon' or 'look good' should not be eaten because you won't be psychologically satisfied by them." People crave what their jaded appetites desire; so how can these types of people be satisfied with any natural, unadulterated, wholesome food?

The Save Your Life Diet (Dr. David Reuben)—An excellent new book discussing the prevention of colon cancer by the daily intake of roughage (in this case bran is lauded). Dr. Reuben gets the credit, but this is not a new discovery. We, in Natural Hygiene, have been belaboring this subject for many years, but it seems to take a "famous authority" before people will listen. There are other books now out on the same subject. Everyone hops on the bandwagon.

Natural Way to Diet—I finally thought someone was on the right track, but I should have known better. Some quotes: "Meat and fish are essential to any diet because you must have proper nutrients." (What is meant by "proper nutrients" in meat and fish? There's no elaboration on it. There are more proper nutrients in food grown from the soil.) Also to quote: "You must have liver since there is no substitute for natural iron." (Pound for pound, there's more iron in sunflower seeds, pumpkin seeds, sesame seeds, and soybeans than there is in beef liver.) These diet books are written by so-called authorities and people come to believe everything they say without question.

Truth About Weight Control (Dr. Neil Solomon)—
Here is another "authority" who has influenced vast numbers of people. This diet is basically like others, although
it does recommend "moderation and balance as keynotes
to good nutrition" and no alcohol or salt, basically no
desserts (with some exceptions), and the use of raw vegetables for emergency craving. For dessert, such things as
caviar, smoked salmon, squab, and pheasant are recommended by Dr. Solomon. He believes in F.M.S. (fat mo-
bilizing substance) to keep weight off permanently. This
F.M.S. is found in the urine of fasting persons. He talks
about "starvation" diets, completely unaware of the difference between fasting and starving. There's a section
that describes how extremely obese husbands and wives
can lose 100 to 150 calories by mastering several types
of sex acts which require various vigorous reciprocal
motions. Who cares?

For the *Yo Yo Test Diet* are recommended: bacon
(loaded with salt), coffee three times a day (increases
fatty acid level of the blood, among other things), white
bread, hot dogs, ice cream, margarine (made from hydrogenated oils). These are abominations. My section on
"food additives" will clarify many of these things.

Solomon says, "Children, from infancy on, should be
taught good eating habits and basic nutrition and . . .
eating habits of small children are largely developed in
the home environment," yet does not indicate what are
good eating habits and basic nutrition.

A strict three-meal-a-day, no-in-between-snacks diet is
mentioned, but what is it? Also mentioned is a "well-
balanced diet," but what is it?

Dr. Solomon's Easy, No-Risk Diet—Quote: "Imagine

being able to eat pretzels, ice cream, or chocolate chip cookies and not feel you're cheating! You will also experience the comfort of knowing you are on a diet that is nutritious, healthy and free of risks to your body. . . ." Dr. Solomon condemns the use of salt, yet allows bacon, green olives, dill pickles, ham, etc., and says that vegetables should be cooked in salted water. Allows "diet" sodas, including colas (contain caffeine), up to 24 ounces (two bottles) a day. On days when four to six meals are used, the overtaxed digestive system never gets a chance to rest. It is constantly working, so how can optimum digestion and function be expected to continue? Allows all types of meats, including crab, lobster, oysters and clams (which are the lowest forms of protein because they are scavengers that live off of the garbage of the sea, i.e., fecal and other waste matters; they also contain larger amounts of lead, mercury and other poisons), also cold cuts and hot dogs which are most abundantly loaded with meat by-products (snouts, ears, lips, bladders, udders, etc.) and harmful chemical additives. Allows peanut butter, but does not specify homemade, so it must be commercial, which uses sugar, salt, and the hydrogenation process (as in making margarine and Crisco). Allows many white (chemically bleached) flour products such as bagels, bread, doughnuts, cakes, cookies, waffles, hot dog and hamburger rolls, pop-ups, etc. Allows cooked and dried cereals (which are nutritionally lacking due to commercial processing and exposure to high temperatures), noodles, spaghetti, frozen french fries, rice (doesn't specify brown or natural so it must be devitalized white), saltine crackers, pretzels, pizza, potato chips, cheese tidbits, Fritos, and other "foods" loaded with salt.

Coffee or tea is on the menu three times a day. Recommends various brand name egg substitutes, but the mono- and diglycerides (fats) plus other additives in them are probably more detrimental than the cholesterol in the eggs. Not much emphasis, in the menus, on fresh raw vegetables and fruits. In fact, in some menus they are omitted or negligible or optional. Allows all kinds of ice creams and popsicles (loaded with sugar, chemical flavors, artificial colors, emulsifiers, etc.). Allows sugar, pork sausage links, jelly. A case history is given of a 16-year-old girl who Dr. Solomon says, "eats such *junk-food* favorites as pizza, potato chips, pretzels and the more nutritional but still fattening ice cream." These "foods" are classified by Dr. Solomon, elsewhere in his book, as junk-foods, yet as a part of his various types of *No-Risk Diets* these same "foods" are included. The *Easy, No-Risk Diet* has a list of "Ten Tips from Successful Dieters," and number six states: "Banish all junk-foods from the house." This is typical of the many contradictions that appear throughout the book. Are the results of these contradictions going to help evolve long-lasting vital health? No way! Solomon refers to soda pop as one example of empty calories and he says, "It is something that all dieters should ruthlessly cut out." Yet in his general instructions for his *Easy, No-Risk Diet* he allows up to 24 ounces (two bottles) of diet soda daily. A corn oil margarine is recommended as better than butter. That's fine if the corn oil remained as is; however, the process of hydrogenation not only makes it a saturated fat (which is to be avoided in the first place), but it requires various potentially harmful chemicals to add taste and flavor and to color the axle grease-type mess. If I had my druthers, I'd druther call it an *Easy, High-Risk Diet*.

Sexy Pineapple Diet—I didn't research it, because just the name fascinated me. But if I were to have my way with it, I'd take one pineapple, give it to a hula girl and chase her. When I had caught her I'd throw away the pineapple—or is it vice versa? One could conceivably lose weight through all this action.

I haven't scratched the surface of fad diets, but the few I've mentioned should give you some enlightenment. They are all variations on a theme and I believe they all insist on meat. There is no doubt that one can and usually does lose weight with these. That is their prime purpose. But one thing you can be sure of is that none of the fad diets supply all the needs of the body in the proper form or amounts. These are still the same foods that our "sick" populations have been eating all their lives. Only in fad diets, these foods are used in excessive or insufficient amounts (creating imbalances) and in forms not in the best interest of our bodies (not of the highest order). Fad diets are like games, and since they do not teach us how to evolve optimum health, it stands to reason that if these diets are followed for an indefinite period of time, ill health and diseases can be the eventual result.

One of the biggest dangers to health, particularly to those who do not live on a natural diet, is the ingestion of chemical food additives. In order to sell in a competitive market, food manufacturers must process their food, preserve it for long shelf life, color it an attractive ripe color, sweeten it, emulsify it, cure it, stabilize it, salt it, irradiate it, bleach it, blanch it, polish it, de-germ it, de-bran it, gas it, spray it with insecticides, with nematocides, with rodenticides and fungicides—all added to the sex hormones, antibiotics, tranquilizers, disinfectants, antispoilants, antisprouting agents, desiccants, and sex-sterilants that the animal or plant has been given previously.

By the time some of this processed food reaches your mouth, it is loaded with enough chemicals to start a drug store. Many of these chemicals are of proven high toxicity, some of them carcinogenic (tending to cause cancer), and almost all the rest have been insufficiently tested, and their effects are unknown.

There are probably close to 3,000 or more food additives, of which close to 2,000 are synthetic chemicals, most of which have never been tested for carcinogenicity. We must realize that every poison taken into the body, if not immediately excreted, must be detoxified by the body. This puts a severe burden on the liver in particular and other organs in general. This means the liver must steal vitamins, especially B complex and C, which are essential aids in detoxification. This tends to deplete the body of vitamin security.

The sad but subtle truth is that since there are usually no immediate reactions to the small amounts ingested, it is the hidden cumulative effects that are responsible for much disease and cancer today. Because these poisons appear in the food in small amounts, don't be fooled that they are safe. These small amounts are still the *same* poisons, only the effects are insidious. Don't be lulled into a false sense of security. Doctors today cannot seem to conceive the fact that many diseases in their patients are the results of 10, 15, 20, 30 or more years of accumulated build-up of these "small amounts" of food additives and other types of pollutants within the cell substance of their bodies. In addition, however, as if to add insult to injury and because it cannot seem to be prevented, the government allows commercially prepared and processed foods to contain an "accepted" percentage of dirt, debris, and insect parts. So look a bit closer at that next candy bar, or whatever, and you may be able to spot a little bonus in it for you.

These additives are supposed to be added in the food in so-called safe amounts, but the important fact is that the average person eats a wide variety and abundance of these adulterated foods three or more times each day, seven days a week, 52 weeks, 365 days a year. That would be well over 1,000 meals and snacks containing the "small amounts" of poisons which are accumulating in your body.

Panic in the Pantry is a book written by Drs. Elizabeth Whelan and Frederick Stare. They take issue with everyone (doctors, scientists, citizens, etc.) who might be against chemical additives in foods. To quote: "Eat your additives, they're good for you." They tell you that poisonous additives such as BHT, sodium nitrite, artificial colorings and flavorings, etc., are not only completely safe but important additions to our daily diet and contribute to our physical and psychological well-being. The term "faddist" is used continually throughout the book, which is probably the authors' way of trying to downgrade those of us who don't agree with them even though we are sincerely concerned with our own health and the health of our children. The primary objective seems to be to persuade the people that small amounts of poisons in the form of food additives (flavorings, colorings, preservatives, emulsifiers, stabilizers and bleached white sugar) are not only safe but nutritious. In my opinion, the book is rather subversive and replete with misinformation. Admittedly there are several items which can be agreed upon, but there is just enough truth presented to make it believable. Only an aware reader would know what important facts have been omitted. However, take warning: the naive, uninformed public could easily be misled and lulled into a false sense of security.

Former Secretary of Agriculture Earl Butz delivered an address before the Institute of Food Technologists in Anaheim, California, June 6, 1976. He said, in part, that "If the world's people are to eat as well, or hopefully even better tomorrow than they do today, then the rule of reason is going to have to prevail in the use of food technology. Innovation must not be hampered on this front. This inevitably means the increased use of chemicals on the farm, and new food manufacturing processes in the food industry, i.e., antibiotics, growth regulators, hormones and what have you." Just what is meant by "what have you"?

Secretary Butz went on further to say that various agents used on the farm and in the food industry will be poisonous and dangerous and that some food additives may cause cancer in laboratory animals. He concluded these thoughts with, "We must constantly ask ourselves whether the benefits from carefully controlled use of such agents outweigh the risks." I look at these statements and wonder where we are headed.

Butz makes several misleading conclusions: He says we must use pesticides in farming; he estimates that 50 million people in America would face starvation if we relied solely on organic farming; foods grown in organic soil and without pesticides cost more; natural fertilizer is not superior and makes for deficient crops; there are health risks in natural fertilizers (he uses Korea as an example, implying that we use human wastes as they do—which we do not).

Dr. Barry Commoner, a noted and respected researcher from Washington University in St. Louis, has found that the price of commercial fertilizers has recently doubled; that farmers using organic methods for years found the fertility of their soil had increased. They found that insect problems decreased when they switched to organic methods. The natural predators of the insects returned and controlled them—no pesticides were used. *The New York Times* for July 20, 1975, showed the results of laboratory tests of the crops of organic farmers. The crops contained more protein, essential minerals and trace minerals than the commercially raised crops.

Let me list a few food additives, without making a treatise on the subject, and give you some idea of the inherent dangers of these additives:

Coumarin—Used for 75 years in imitation vanilla before it was found to produce liver damage in animals.

Dulcin—Used for 50 years as a sugar substitute before it was found to produce cancer in animals.

Butter Yellow—A coal-tar derivative used as a food coloring. Has been found to produce cancer of the liver in animals. (As a point of information, any coal-tar derivative is carcinogenic and most of the food additives are coal-tar derivatives.)

Mineral Oil—Was once used in salad dressings and as a substitute for food oils, but was found to interfere with digestion and the absorption of vitamins—mainly vitamin A.

Piperonal—An inexpensive substitute for costly vanilla flavoring. It is used industrially to kill lice.

Butyraldehyde—Used for a nutty flavor. Industrially, it is an ingredient in rubber cement and synthetic resins.

Aldehyde C-17—Used for a cherry taste. It is a flammable liquid used industrially in aniline dyes, plastics, and synthetic rubbers.

Ethyl Acetate—Used for a pineapple flavor. The vapor can cause chronic lung, liver, and heart damage. This chemical is used industrially as a solvent for plastics and lacquers.

Methylcellulose—Thickener used in processed cheese. It is used commercially in cosmetics and adhesives.

Sodium Carboxymethylcellulose—Used as a cheese stabilizer and as a thickener in ice cream and whipped topping mixes. It is found in resin emulsion paints and printing inks. It can cause intestinal obstruction and has produced arterial lesions (diseases in the arteries) similar to high blood cholesterol.

8-Hydroxyquinoline—A former preservative in cottage cheese. This has been found to cause cancer in mice and is used in contraceptives and rectal suppositories.

Alginic Acid—Used in cheese spreads to give uniformity of color and flavor. It is used industrially in making artificial ivory and celluloid.

Benzoyl Peroxide—Used as a bleach in domestic Gorgonzola, Blue, Provolone, Romano, and Parmesan cheeses. This chemical destroys every trace of vitamin A.

Resinous Glaze—An innocent term for a shellac which gives polish or glaze to candies, such as chocolate-covered raisins, etc. There is also another type of resinous glaze which is obtained from certain insect secretions in the West Indies.

PVP (polyvinylpyrrolidone)—Used in beer for clarity and is being tested for use in wines, fruit juices, and jellies. This chemical is also used in aerosol hair sprays.

Coal-Tar Derivative Paraffin—Coats fresh fruits and vegetables to prevent spoilage.

Beta-Naphthylamine—This is used to make two coal-tar dyes to color butter and oleomargarine. Has caused bladder cancer in animals.

Calcium or Sodium Propionate—Retards molding and spoilage in breads; it is a fungicide. I have used this chemical in my practice and have gotten good results in the treatment of athlete's foot.

Chicle—Is a latex rubber used in chewing gum. Chewing gum also contains antioxidants, synthetic flavors, and colors which are coal-tar derivatives.

Calcium Chloride—Used in cheesemaking to set the milk in a semisolid mass, and in canned potatoes, lima beans, tomatoes, etc., to keep them firm or crisp. It is also used in the canning of milk to adjust the salt balance and prevent curdling. This chemical is used to melt snow and to oil down dusty roads and can cause metal parts to disintegrate. Can cause stomach irritation and kidney impairment.

Sodium Citrate or Phosphate—This is also used in the canning of milk, but can aggravate an already high blood pressure.

Magnesium Carbonate—Used in bleaching cheese and also to keep the green color in canned vegetables. Other uses are as a powerful laxative, for fireproofing wood, in disinfectants, and in manufacturing cotton fabrics.

Acetic Acid—Used as a dip for shrimp and other fish meats to prevent discoloration. It is also used in the manufacturing of plastics and dyeing of silks. I have used it in a concentrated form for the removal of warts.

Chlorine Dioxide—A dangerous toxic explosive gas, one good whiff of which will render you *non compos mentis*. This is used to bleach the flour which goes into white bread, etc. It destroys vitamin E, among other things.

Brominated Vegetable Oils—Used in soft drinks for uniform distribution of fruity flavors. This has shown evidence of inducing damage in the liver, heart, thyroid, and kidneys of rats and interferes with normal fat metabolism.

Stearic Acid—A white crystalline fatty acid, usually extracted from tallow and other hard fats. Used in making cosmetics, soaps, suppositories, and pill coatings.

Mesityl Oxide—Used for color and flavor. This is a petroleum-based compound found in lubricating oils, insecticides, plastic wrapping material, can linings, adhesives, inks, and varnishes. It has the characteristic odor of the urine of tomcats and is sometimes detected in some of the plastic food wrapping material you might have around the house.

Sodium Benzoate—A deadly poison used as a preservative in soda pop, jams, jellies, pickles, and countless other so-called foods. Speaking of soda, caffeine is used in all cola drinks. The concerned parent who forbids the child the ingestion of coffee or tea unknowingly allows the child to consume enormous amounts of caffeine when the unlimited use of cola drinks is permitted. Sodium

Benzoate kills or inhibits all living organisms present within the jar or other container. We are living organisms too, but the harmful effects, because of the small doses in food products, don't make themselves evident until years later, except in those cases of frank sensitivity which can result in a severe reaction and/or death. (This applies to any of the myriad of chemical additives.)

Sulfur Dioxide—Used in processing sugar and as a bacterial inhibitor in wines, imitation jelly, beverages, etc. Also used as a bleaching agent for many foods, such as nuts in shells, sliced potatoes used for French fries, figs and other fruits. Additional sulfur dioxide gets into our systems as we breathe it from the air, since it is a major pollutant from factories. It is a proven poison. It has been found to increase uric acid, to produce inflammation of the mucous membranes of the mouth, to cause nausea, anemia, malaise, etc. Sulfur dioxide can produce cancer and interfere with cell function (as most of these poisons can). Drs. Braverman and Shapiro (biochemists) reported that when a form of sulfur dioxide is applied to a component of nucleic acid, the basic unit of heredity, then the component Uracil is unable to perform its usual function. These findings have raised questions on the long-range possibility of genetic damage.

Polyoxyethylene Compounds—Used as a replacement for natural shortenings and as an emulsifier in breads and reduces the quantity needed of natural ingredients. It increases the volume of foods and is found also in biscuits, cake mixes, ice cream, frozen desserts, pickles, etc. Has also been used in tobacco to retain moisture, but caused bladder stones and tumors in experimental rats and was taken out. It has been found to cause easier absorption of pesticide residues, gastrointestinal irritation, changes in intestinal flora (beneficial bacteria), hives and disturbances in bile secretions.

DES (diethylstilbestrol)—A synthetic female sex hormone which cheaply puts weight, fat, and water on cattle and poultry. This is one of the most dangerous of additives. In human beings, it has produced breast cancer, fibroid tumors of the uterus, excessive menstrual bleeding, sterility and impotence in men and arrested growth in children. Current research has found evidence of vaginal cancer in the daughters of mothers who had taken DES, also a relationship of cancer of the prostate in male offspring of mothers who had taken DES.

Hydrogenated Oil—Prevents rancidity and deterioration in commercial peanut butters and scores of processed foods and candies. It alters the biological qualities in food. In this case, the vegetable oil is subjected to an extremely high temperature and in the presence of a metal catalyst such as nickel or platinum, hydrogen gas is bubbled through the oil, causing its saturation or hardening. The result is a smelly, axle grease-like mess that has to be bleached, filtered, and deodorized. All of the essential fatty acids in the original oil are destroyed.

Disodium EDTA—Used to promote color, flavor, and texture retention in canned carbonated soft drinks, distilled alcoholic beverages, vinegar, canned white potatoes, clams, crabmeat, and shrimp. Also in cooked canned mushrooms, various canned beans, pickled cucumbers and cabbage, and in liquid multi-vitamin preparations. It is also used in beer, mayonnaise, margarine, potato salad, and sandwich spreads, etc. In the human body, it inhibits enzymes and blood coagulation, causes gastrointestinal disturbances, muscle cramps, and kidney damage. It can also combine with calcium, iron, and other nutrients and prevent them from being utilized by the body, since it is used for trapping metal impurities in foods. The potential hazards of this food additive, as with others, are the small quantities ingested in a variety of foods and beverages daily over a long period of time.

Butylated Hydroxyanisole (BHA) and Butylated Hydroxytoluene (BHT)—These are two of the most widely used antioxidants in foods, which stabilize fats so they don't become rancid due to their loss of natural antioxidants in factory processing. BHA is in almost every processed food that the "average person" eats. I can't begin to list the endless names of the foods. BHT is used in as many foods as BHA. For example: cereals, rice, shortenings, potato flakes, sugar, cured meats, potato chips, etc. These two chemicals are also used in making plastic packaging material, rubber gaskets, milk cartons, wax paper, and lubricants. Both have caused dermatitis (skin disease), severe allergic reactions such as disabling chronic asthmatic attacks, skin blistering, eye hemorrhaging, tingling of face and hands, extreme weakness and fatigue, edema (swelling), chest tightness, and difficulty in breathing.

Propylene Glycol—A stabilizer used in ice cream, candies, synthetic whipped toppings and in almost everything processed that the "average person" eats. This chemical is used in germicides, paint removers and antifreeze substances. Propylene glycol always reminds me of the time, a number of years ago, when my youngest son was admitted to the hospital for a hernia repair. We requested a vegetarian diet for him and argued with the powers-that-be just to get simple unprocessed, uncanned fresh fruits and vegetables. Evidently the entire idea was over their heads and we brought in our own food. The point is that on each tray that was brought at mealtimes was a disposable, individually wrapped germicidal hand-wipe. One of the ingredients was propylene glycol and, ironically, almost every tray had some type of packaged, processed food product (synthetic or otherwise) which contained propylene glycol as a preservative. We threw it out each time.

Red Dye No. 2 (Amaranth)—One of the many coal tar dyes; but this one has gained universal acceptance. Principal uses have been in beverages, but it is also widely used in candy, confections, pet food, dessert powders, bakery goods, sausages, ice cream, sherbet, dairy products, cereals, snack foods, etc. Allergists have reported cases of Amaranth sensitivity. The Russians have done extensive research on this synthetic food coloring and have found that it not only tends to produce cancer, but could cause malformed and softened fetuses (unborn babies). It was finally banned in 1976; however, it is supposed to be replaced by Red Dye No. 40, which is as bad or worse than Red Dye No. 2.

Sodium Nitrate and Sodium Nitrite—There is probably almost no one who hasn't taken these chemicals into his body and most people ingest them on a daily basis. Used as a preservative and color fixative in cured meats, meat products, and certain cured fish, such as bacon, bologna, hot dogs, deviled ham, meat spreads, potted meats, almost all ham, sausages, smoked and cured shad, salmon, tuna fish products, poultry, wild game, pickled corned beef, tongue, pastrami, and a host of cold cuts. Meats, no matter in what stage of decay, are kept a pinkish color, which implies freshness. If most of the meats did not have these two chemicals within, most people would probably not buy the product, since it would resemble a gray, colorless cadaver (corpse). The danger is that sodium nitrite tends to lessen the blood's ability to carry oxygen and if ingested in sufficient quantities can lead to respiratory failure. Recent studies at the Children's Cancer Research Foundation showed that the nitrites can cause cancer, can be mutagenic (causing changes in the form of an individual due to a change in the genes or chromosomes), teratogenic (causing monstrosities), and generally toxic (poisonous) to the entire human system. Sodium nitrate tends to neutralize and is antagonistic to vitamin A. It becomes more troublesome when intestinal bacteria convert it to sodium nitrite. A class of compounds termed nitrosamines is one of the most powerful cancer-producing agents known to science according to Drs. Samuel Epstein and William Lijinsky of the Children's Cancer Research Foundation and University of Nebraska's College of Medicine, respectively. Nitrosamines are present in many food materials and have been shown to act throughout the body and produce cancer in a wide range of organs and species. Nitrates and nitrites in some foods can combine in the digestive tract with secondary amines, which are also present in some foods. Under certain circumstances, this combining can produce nitrosamines which are potential cancer-producing compounds.

I hope this brief presentation will open your eyes and your minds and make you more aware of the possible hazards of eating foods other that what grows from the ground in their fresh, unadulterated state. Be wary of any commercially processed foods. The choice is yours. You now have some basic tools with which to make decisions —decisions which can affect the rest of your life and the lives of your children.

There are many books published on food additives which you can obtain to further enhance your knowledge; but the next time you shop in a supermarket, read the labels. Read labels on everything you can and you'll get an education in pharmaceutics.

CHAPTER **X**

Natural Living—Where It's At!

The American Natural Hygiene Society, with head-quarters at 1920 Irving Park Road, Chicago, Illinois 60613, is a non-profit, non-sectarian educational organization which promotes the knowledge of natural living as a means of maintaining and restoring health. Ironically, the philosophy of Natural Hygiene was evolved mostly by medical doctors, almost 150 years ago, who found their medical practices an incorrect approach to health care. These medical men reasoned that there were natural laws which governed human life and that when these laws were applied, health could be both maintained and recovered.

"Hygiene" is derived from the Greek "hygieia," referring to the science of health. Natural Hygiene is that branch of biological science which studies, investigates, and applies the conditions upon which life and health depend. It teaches that health and disease are not the results of chance, but depend upon the operation of certain demonstrable laws. Natural Hygiene studies and attempts to understand the influence of air, water, food, sunshine, activity, exercise, rest, sleep, fasting, mental and emotional factors, etc. It represents a comprehensive system

—a way of life in harmony with natural laws as they apply to man.

There are many books on the subject of Natural Hygiene, which will be listed later for the broadening of your knowledge. This final chapter will give you the basics so you will have a working understanding from which to gain a deeper insight. I want to plant the seeds of this philosophy into your mind in hopes they will take root and grow.

When we view the living being down at the cell level, we find two basic requirements of life as all-important: (1) adequate and complete nourishment, and (2) prompt and thorough removal of all metabolic waste. (Metabolism is the total of the body processes which keep it alive, nourished, and functioning.) Without both of these requirements being fulfilled, life would cease.

Most disease is the result of enervation. Enervation is lowered nerve energy, which in turn lowers functioning power. When enervation is present, elimination of metabolic waste is impaired. (Our billions and billions of cells are constantly giving off waste products. If they did not, then we would die.) This impairment of elimination of these metabolic wastes results in our bodily tissues being poisoned by the retention and accumulation of its own cell wastes. This is called toxemia. Enervation may occur for many reasons, all of which tax the body: overwork; overeating; lack of fresh air; sexual excesses (some will argue this point); excessive bathing; too much sun; lack of rest and sleep; lack of exercise; lack of adequate food; too much or too little of any good thing; lack of emotional poise, resulting in fear, hate, worry and anger; the use of harmful elements such as coffee, tea, alcohol, tobacco, chocolate, drugs, etc.; also various environmental stresses. In consequence, this is the very beginning of a pathological process which can lead to cancer. The first step is of course, *enervation*. This is followed by the second step, *toxemia*. This progresses to *inflammation* or *irritation*. It is these initial three steps which are usually missed by the doctor, since he is basically unaware of the sequence of events in the evolution of disease. Thus, most people are usually well into disease, where frank damage is already done, before the doctor finally sees "something." The fourth step is *ulceration*, which leads to the fifth step, *fibrosis* (hardening with fibrous tissue). The sixth step, of course, is *cancer*.

One of the most misunderstood of conditions is the "common cold." It seems scientists and doctors are searching for the ever-evasive virus which is supposed to cause it. What is a "cold"? It is nothing more than the body ridding itself of its toxic load so it does not build up in the system to cause more serious and debilitating problems. This is why all the mucous membranes are involved (nose, throat, lungs, intestines, etc.). These membranes are eliminating the toxic materials. Many times, these viruses thrive in this medium and can complicate the condition—but secondarily, and usually in an unhealthy individual. A cold is *a vital capacity*, the body's effort to cleanse itself. How many times have you heard someone remark about "so and so" was only 45 or 50 years old, never had a sick day in his life, and suddenly dropped dead from a heart attack. If "so and so" might have gotten a few colds, he might not have had that heart attack. He didn't die suddenly. He was dying for years.

I observe old people in convalescent homes. There's

much pride there when it is shown that "they don't get colds." Of course they don't! Most of them do not have the vital capacity to get a cold. So this build-up in the body (toxemia or self-poisoning) of metabolic waste, etc., manifests itself in other ways, such as the chronic, debilitating diseases most of them are vegetating from, and to which many of them succumb.

Be thankful when you get a cold. Rest in bed, fast a few days just drinking water (or take small amounts of fresh-made fruit juices and preferably vegetable juices if you must). Don't suppress the fever with aspirin; the fever is remedial. Don't suppress the symptoms with various drugs. This is why complications occur, such as pneumonia, because the body is always interfered with. In fact, much disease is remedial, but continual interference with drugs prolongs the disease or complicates matters, and when the body gets well, it gets well not because of the drugs or medicines, but in spite of them.

Natural Hygiene is a plan of living which, briefly, is comprised of such things as the use of pure water; breathing pure air; maintenance of emotional poise; getting plenty of sunshine and rest; the avoidance of anything harmful to the body, such as coffee, tea, alcohol, tobacco, chocolate, white sugar, white flour, salt, meat, drugs and medicines, chemical food additives, soda, canned and processed foods, etc. Also included is proper use of exercise (depending on one's physical limitations), vegetarian diet (but if a completely meatless diet is not your choice, there is still a great deal to learn about how to improve your present diet and state of health and health of your family), and of course the all-important fast.

All infants are, with few exceptions, born with a natural immunity and resistance which are further enhanced by breast feeding. But since so many young mothers are discouraged from breast feeding and encouraged to use formulas and not given a knowledge of proper nutrition, this is how these natural immunities and resistances become lowered and the infant becomes the "average" child who gets the usual childhood diseases and worse. He (or she) is fed the usual diet of mostly cooked, processed, and devitalized foods. Baby cereal (starch) is fed in infancy when there is no capacity to digest this starch, so it putrefies and the infant is virtually poisoned by it in addition to acquiring colic and spitting up. Until the infant gets his teeth to chew and properly insalivate the starch, he should not be fed any. In so-called backward countries, when the infant is to be fed a starch, the innate wisdom of the mother induces her to chew it thoroughly and mix it with her saliva and pre-digest it (her saliva has the enzyme ptyalin for starch breakdown) before putting it into the infant's mouth.

The juicer and blender become most valuable assets because fresh fruit and vegetable juices can be made with the juicer, while with the blender, pure and unadulterated baby food (both raw and cooked) can be made from fresh fruits and vegetables. My wife has often confided to me that if I were to write a book on the proper nutrition of children, she would want me to trace much of the illness today back to the kitchen of "good old mom," because it is basically her responsibility and obligation.

I would like to elaborate on two phases of Natural Hygiene so you will have a clearer understanding of what appears to be unorthodox and controversial only because of misunderstandings and closed-mindedness, yet are as natural and physiologically sound as any laws of nature can be: (1) fasting, and (2) proper nutrition and food combining.

Fasting is complete and total abstinence from all food, with the exception of water, where the body supports itself on the stored reserves within its tissues. It is important to make the differentiation between fasting and starvation, because many people use these two terms interchangeably in error. Starvation begins when the fast is carried beyond the time when these stored reserves are used up or have dropped to a dangerously low level and the vital organs begin to be consumed by the body for food, and death becomes imminent.

There are several reasons for fasting: (1) Weight reduction. In cases of overweight individuals, weight reduction is an added benefit even when not the sole or even the main reason for the fast; (2) To conserve the energies of the body so they may be diverted to whatever the body is trying to accomplish; (3) To secure physiologic rest. This is rest of the digestive, glandular, circulatory, respiratory, and nervous systems. It is during this physiologic rest (fasting) that the body is able to repair its damaged organs; and, (4) Elimination. Nothing known to man equals the fast as a means of increasing the elimination of waste from the blood and tissues. As the fast continues and more of the toxic load is thrown out, the system becomes purified and one improves health or recovers health.

There are three important facts to note: (1) Because of its intracellular (within the cells) enzymes, the body is capable of digestion of its own proteins, fats, and carbohydrates; (2) The body is fully capable of controlling the self-digesting process (autolysis) and rigidly limits it to nonessential and less essential tissues. Even in starvation, when the vital tissues begin to be consumed, there is rigid control as these tissues are drawn upon in an inverse proportion to their relative importance; and (3) The body is capable of utilizing the end products of this autolytic (self) disintegration to nourish its most vital and most essential parts.

Water is lost first. Energy first comes from combustion of carbohydrates, then fat reserves, then tissue protein. Even after a prolonged fast, nitrogen excretion shows a pronounced fall, the nitrogen being retained for reconstruction of tissue protein. The nitrogen excreted early in the fast is derived from the mobilization of reserve protein. The excretion of sodium, potassium, calcium, and other minerals is reduced after the first few days of fasting, and normal blood levels are then maintained showing evidence that they are conserved.

The body regenerates itself constantly and the daily renewal of its cells and tissues prevents old age and death for a considerable time in spite of abuses committed against it. The process of regeneration stays ahead of the process of degeneration as a result of fasting, so a higher level of health is thus reached. Man cannot live for many generations or shrink down and then grow into a young man, but there is, to an extent, a renewal of man's body.

Hawk, Oser, and Summerson state: "Abstinence from food for a short time can in no way operate to the disadvantage of a normal person. In fact, individuals affected with certain types of gastrointestinal disorders are benefitted by fasting. Fasting has also been used in cases of diabetes and obesity."

Fasts of long duration (beyond four or five days to a week) should be properly supervised by competent professional hygienic practitioners (be they medical, osteopathic, or chiropractic physicians). It is vitally important to break a long fast correctly to avoid any potential hazards to the body. Fasting is virtually safe if handled properly, particularly when you compare the fact that there are over 100,000 deaths a year due to the taking of prescription drugs, according to Drs. Milton Silverman and Philip Lee (researchers) of the University of California at San Francisco (UCSF).

There are some contraindications to fasting: (1) Fear of the fast; (2) Extreme emaciation. Sometimes a short fast of one to three days or a series of short fasts with intervals of proper feeding are beneficial; (3) Extreme weakness or degeneration. In late or terminal cancer the only value is that fasting will relieve the patient's suffering and allow him to die in relative peace rather than in severe pain as a narcotics addict. Regarding cancer, I remember a prominent physician stating that "the single most important need is early detection." I must disagree with that because early detection means the person already has cancer. I believe the single most important need is *prevention,* whether it be for cancer or any other disease. George Crile, M.D., uses the term starvation instead of fasting, but he states: "It is in selective starvation that one of the great hopes for the future lies. It is possible that ultimately cancer will be controlled not by attacking the cancer, but by starving it or by altering the environment in which it lives"; (4) Severe deficiency disease. The person should be built up with proper diet before a fast is attempted; (5) Sometimes with difficult breathing, as in heart cases and should heart action weaken, the fast should be terminated; and (6) Pregnancy. Lactating mothers should not fast.

As one gets into a fast, certain developments occur almost like clockwork: The tongue becomes coated, the breath and taste become foul, and the teeth become pasty. This is due to the body's unloading of its toxic burden. Almost automatically, after the third day, true hunger and sincere desire for food subside and you become quite comfortable. As long as this hunger is absent, it indicates that no food is required. However, one of the main indications for terminating the fast is the return of true hunger. This is the body's inner wisdom in action, preventing the entering of the starvation period. An interesting fact is that most people have never really experienced and enjoyed true hunger. True hunger is a comfortable mouth and throat sensation, as is thirst. The "average" person experiences what is termed "hunger pangs" or gnawing in the stomach. This is a morbid sensation—not a normal indication of hunger. The years of overeating, smoking, drinking, the use of salt and other irritants and/or poisons, etc., contribute to this abnormal sensation of hunger which is nothing more than irritation (the earliest warning sign of impending and incipient ulcer and, in some cases, cancer). This inner wisdom is always at work for us, but most people ignore or are completely unaware of it. The so-called "dumb" animal is aware—why aren't we? Observe your pet dog or cat who is supposed to be less intelligent than the human. He doesn't know about drugs, medicines, or doctors. Yet, what does he do when he doesn't feel well? He fasts! Other indications for breaking the fast are that the foul breath and taste become sweet and clean, the heavily coated tongue becomes pink and clear, salivary secretion becomes normal (it usually is thicker and in smaller quantities during a fast), the temperature, which may have been subnormal, returns to normal and the usually dark and odorous urine becomes light and loses its strong odor.

Contrary to misbeliefs and old wives' tales, fasting does not cause the stomach to atrophy (wither and become useless) or its walls to adhere or its digestive fluids to turn upon itself and digest it, does not paralyze the bowels, does not deplete the blood or produce anemia, does not produce an acidosis that results in death, does not cause the heart to weaken or collapse, does not produce deficiency or malnutritional disease and its edema (swelling), does not reduce resistance to disease, does not harm the teeth, the nervous system, glands or vital organs, does not weaken the vital powers or cause mental disturbances. Blood sugar is little depressed; it is synthesized from protein.

Fasting, itself, does not cure disease. It gives the body the environment to heal itself—physiologic rest. However, this is what fasting does do: (1) It gives the vital organs a complete rest; (2) It stops the intake of foods that decompose in the intestines and further poison the body; (3) It promotes elimination of metabolic wastes; (4) It allows the body to adjust and normalize its biochemistry and also its secretions (glandular fluids); (5) It lets the body break down and absorb swellings, deposits, diseased tissues, and abnormal growths; (6) It restores a youthful condition to the cells and tissues and in a relative sense rejuvenates the body; (7) It permits the conservation and re-routing of energy; (8) It increases the powers of digestion and assimilation (absorption and utilization of food into the system); (9) It clears and strengthens the mind; and (10) It improves function throughout the body. Of course, if there are irreversible changes, the results may be poor to none.

Actually, the fast will have been in vain if the individual returns to his old habits, and the results will be more or less temporary. Fasting does not make one disease-proof. Hygienic living is essential after the fast if good health is to be the continued and permanent result.

Fasting is a means to an end. It is a cleansing process and a physiologic or functional rest which prepares the body for future correct living.

In his book, *Fasting: The Ultimate Diet* (a worthy contribution on the subject of fasting), Dr. Allan Cott recommends: (1) "Drink at least two quarts of water every day"; (2) "If the object of your fast is to lose weight, you will lose it that much more quickly by adhering to a daily exercise program"; and (3) "Exercise as much as you can."

It is important, to avoid a potential and very real danger, that these recommendations be re-evaluated and put in a proper perspective: (1) Setting a goal of two quarts or more of water every day is not in harmony with normal physiology. In fact, it is a forcing measure which may cause a mineral imbalance (depletion) from too much flushing of the system with water. Nothing should be forced, whether fasting or not. The body with its innate wisdom will indicate when to drink, when not to drink, and also how much to drink. One should use his or her body's own wisdom as a guide. (During each of my long fasts, I drank *only* when I was thirsty; some days I drank two glasses of water, and some days I consumed two quarts.) Excesses enervate the body, particularly the fasting body, and put more of a burden on it. (2) Regarding Dr. Cott's recommendation of a daily exercise program to lose weight more quickly while fasting, there's an old adage in biochemistry which says, "Fat burns in the flame of carbohydrate." Glucose is a refined carbohydrate. It stands to reason that if the body's supply of glucose is conserved and not depleted through physical exercise, fat will burn more efficiently and thus more weight will be lost while fasting. This is seen regularly at the various natural hygiene institutions. Guests are usually advised to rest after the second day of fasting. This holds true particularly during fasts of longer durations. Some have tried it both ways and agree that resting while fasting produces more beneficial results as well as a more rapid weight loss. (3) My biggest concern is the statement to "exercise as much as you can," which Dr. Cott recommends during fasting. Some of the crises which take place during a fast are due to the side effects of drugs being disengaged from the fat tissues. When one is fasting, the release of deep-seated toxins takes place because of energy from glucose. However, when exercise is carried out, glucose is diverted to the muscles and can cause a hypoglycemia (low blood sugar). This low glucose doesn't give the body enough energy to eliminate the deep-seated toxins. This is the reason why so many people boast of how they can fast for two or three weeks working all the time. The body must expend energy for this work, and the elimination of metabolic wastes and other poisons are hindered. If these people were to lie in bed and rest while fasting, they would eliminate much more efficiently and would undergo these healing crises, which would make them temporarily too "sick" to get out of bed for a while. The body retraces while in a long fast and toxins from past years are eventually thrown out. You might compare this to a thermometer which, as the mercury rises, passes through various gradations; as the mercury falls, it passes back through these gradations.

To clarify and help you further understand this very important point, let us remember that when one is fasting, enzymic functions (specific biochemical reactions) are carried out at a high level of energy. Fuel for energy is supplied by glucose. When no food is being taken into the system, no glucose is being manufactured. Therefore, stored reserves of glucose, taken mainly from the liver and muscles are being utilized. When these reserves begin to diminish, nervous and chemical energy are expended to replace the glucose.

During the fast, glucose is needed to supply energy to effect the carrying off of wastes from the bloodstream and to burn up fat. This same energy, supplied by glucose, is utilized to effect the process of desalination (removal of salt from fatty tissue) which occurs during fasting. Inorganic salt, which the body in its wisdom has mobilized by conjugating it with fat, is now disengaged from the fat and cast into the bloodstream where it is carried basically to the main organ of elimination, the kidneys, which void it.

Glucose aids the buffer systems of the blood to help neutralize the acidity which occurs during the fast. The brain, which uses glucose for fuel, must also be supplied with this vital substance by the bloodstream.

When you are physically active during the fast, glucose (which would be utilized to supply energy for the removal of toxins and metabolic wastes, for the metabolism of fat, for desalination, to fuel the brain, etc.) must be diverted to provide the energy required for physical activity. The result could be a less efficient removal of wastes, a reduction in the amount of fat metabolized, reduced efficiency in the desalination process, and a dangerously low glucose level in the brain. It could cause acidosis because of too concentrated a level of toxins remaining in the bloodstream rather than being excreted efficiently; it could cause rapid heartbeat; it could affect the respiratory center of the brain, causing fainting or a lack of proper breathing. The condition is known as hypoglycemia or low blood sugar.

In an article in the *Journal of the American Medical Association*, November 16, 1963, Dr. Walter Bloom of the Piedmont Hospital in Atlanta, Georgia, states: "Fasting is well tolerated for long periods of time, provided energy expenditure is restricted."

A most important point, regarding exercise during fasting, to also consider is that the body in the fasting state is resting, and the use of exercise may put an excessive strain on the heart and other organs, with life-threatening consequences.

Today we do not stress so much the length of the fast as its effectiveness. To arbitrarily limit the duration of the fast is to limit the benefits one may derive from it. The only logical plan of determining the length of a fast is to watch day-by-day developments and to break or continue the fast according to these. No man possesses sufficient knowledge to determine in advance how much fasting one requires in one's particular condition. In adjusting the length of the fast to individual needs, a close study and observation of the faster, as the fast progresses, is required.

The second phase of Natural Hygiene I'd like to familiarize you with is proper nutrition and food combining. Let us not be confused with the terms nutrition and food. These are not synonymous. It is one thing to have good nutrition, but it is another thing to eat an abundance of food. You are not nourished by the amount of food you eat, but in proportion to the amount you digest and assimilate (absorb and convert into living tissue). The key is assimilation.

According to the research of Dr. Joseph Sasaki, an eminent eye specialist from Ann Arbor, Michigan, many people are not receiving the proper nutrition from their foods because of one important factor—close work during and/or after eating. It is a known physiologic fact that close work, during or immediately after eating hinders digestion and inhibits the proper absorption and assimilation of vitamins B and C and amino acids. This predisposes most human beings to many consequential diseases, in addition to tenseness and nervousness. In fact, many people's tenseness and nervousness have disappeared when close work during and/or after eating was stopped. The problem is that people spend a majority of their time indoors, at home or work, and rarely do they allow their eyes to relax at infinity (beyond 20 feet). Therefore, don't read or watch television during mealtimes; don't read or watch television for one and one-half to two hours after eating; don't close your eyes (as in napping) after eating, since this is the same as doing close work; and don't stay indoors because rarely do you see beyond 20 feet, but if you must, then sit and look out the window into the distance.

Many people do not have the capacity to properly digest and assimilate their food, yet I've seen countless numbers stuffed on all types of foods, particularly protein and fattening food. This stuffing regimen, which is so common, only enervates and further weakens those people who lack the capacity to digest and assimilate. They are similar to people who are anemic and taking iron without improving, or those taking any other so-called food supplements for whatever is supposed to be lacking and yet not getting better. After these methods have failed, stimulants and tonics are usually added. These cannot enhance digestive and assimilative powers, so the individual may become thinner, weaker, and sicker. This is what happened to me as I ran this same gamut during the course of my nightmarish illness. Capacity cannot be bought. There are no drugs that can increase this capacity or carry on our life functions for us. Nothing from any source outside the body can add to its nutritive capacities or healing abilities. Furthermore, if medicines are supposed to make sick people well, then it certainly should be beneficial or harmless for healthy people to take them. So why are they forbidden?

It is as important to know when to abstain from food as it is to know when and how much to eat. There is no benefit derived by eating when no food is required or when food cannot be digested and assimilated. Just as a large pile of bricks does not increase the productive capacity of the bricklayer, so a large supply of food does not increase the digestive and assimilative capacities of the invalid. Fasting, under certain circumstances and conditions, is one way to increase these powers. Generally speaking, the average person should fast 36 hours (a day and a half) a week. For example, eat the last meal on Sunday night; then eat the next meal on Tuesday morning.

In Natural Hygiene, a vegetarian diet is followed, although some people in a transition period or for personal reasons do use occasional meat or fish until they are able to eliminate them. The diet consists mainly of fresh vegetables, fruits, nuts, seeds, and sprouts which are eaten, for the most part, unfired—raw. Some prefer to use a little natural cheese, while some prefer to add some cooked food such as steamed potatoes, brown rice, and a wide variety of very interesting and palate-teasing vegetarian recipes. These foods supply the richest source of minerals, vitamins, and enzymes when eaten raw. Heat (cooking) destroys the enzymes, certain vitamins, and in general the life in the food. Many people maintain they can't handle raw foods. I couldn't either, but after a fast to let the digestive apparatus heal itself, I'm living on foods my doctors said I could never eat again. So it is with others, which indicates that a fast may be necessary.

The present-day diet of Americans is largely denatured. It is made up of white bread, white rice, demineralized cereal grains, pasteurized milk, white sugar, canned fruits and vegetables, cakes, pies, and thoroughly cooked food, all eaten in abominable combinations. There is also the unlimited use of other harmful "foods" such as salt, condiments, coffee, tea, deep-fried foods, alcoholic beverages, pastas (spaghetti, macaroni, etc.), food substitutes (i.e., egg substitutes, non-dairy creamers, etc.), and an endless list of items which denote "gracious living." I have always said that man will eat almost anything, even if it makes him sick or kills him. In fact, if I took some shoe leather, softened it, spiced it as a gourmet would and baked it, I venture to say that someone would eat it. The motto seems to be, "If it tastes good—eat it." People have forgotten the taste of plain, wholesome, natural food.

White sugar is probably responsible for more damage to the mind and body than any other single food-type element. It raises blood cortisone, increases triglycerides (fats) and cholesterol, raises blood uric acid (which can cause gouty arthritis among other things), and increases hydrochloric acid in the stomach. There is no nutriment in white sugar (which is contained in most commercial foods today and has a strong affinity for calcium—so much so that it upsets the calcium-phosphorus balance, which can be serious in a growing child). White sugar can produce hypoglycemia (low blood sugar) because of the constant stimulation of the pancreas to produce insulin in such amounts as to cause a tremendous drop in the blood sugar level. Hyperkinetic (hyperactive) children, according to the latest research, have been found to ingest large amounts of white sugar and chemical food additives; when these were taken away from them, they ceased to be hyperkinetic.

Milk also has no place in the adult diet, since the stomach enzyme rennin, which is responsible for coagulating the milk, is diminished or lacking, thereby making the milk very difficult to digest properly. This is why a natural cheese would be better because it is already coagulated. Pasteurization alters enzymes and vitamins and also destroys an important amino acid (protein building block)—lysine. Then vitamins are artificially added back. Milk is an insulator and when taken with meals retards gastric (stomach) digestion. Another interesting fact is that many children who are anemic are big milk drinkers. Why? Because when they fill up on milk, which has no iron, it prevents them from eating a proper diet which would contain adequate iron. According to the U.S. Department of Agriculture Handbook No. 8, there are many vegetables that contain two to ten times the amount of calcium as milk. There are also those that contain more iron than liver, such as seeds.

There seems to me much concern about pernicious anemia in people who don't eat animal products, particularly vegetarians. The fact is that anyone can suffer a nutritional imbalance through ignorance, neglect, or as a result of the fast pace of living. Doctors' offices are full of people with pernicious anemia, almost all of whom eat meat and other animal products.

Best and Taylor state: "The extrinsic factor (vitamin B-12) is present in liver, beef, rice polishings, yeast, and other substances rich in the vitamin B complex. It is also found in the intestinal contents of normal persons as well as in the feces of patients with pernicious anemia. There is, therefore, no reason to believe that a dietary deficiency of this factor is the cause of the disease. The basic defect in pernicious anemia is the failure of the gastric mucosa (stomach lining or membrane) to produce, at least in effective amounts, the intrinsic factor. It is now believed that this factor is essential for the adequate absorption of vitamin B-12."

I only mention a few foods to give you an idea of why the average person does not have a high degree of health.

It is not in the scope of this book to analyze every food, but there is an important fact about raw natural foods (roughage). Drs. David Kritchevsky and Baruch Modan, of the Wistar Institute in Philadelphia and Johns Hopkins Medical School, respectively, have done research on plant fiber (roughage) and colon cancer. It was found that people who ate a large amount of plant fiber—raw, fresh fruits and vegetables—had a lower incidence of colon cancer. This "roughage," which is indigestible, stimulates the colon to get rid of its contents faster, and as this food moves through the small and lower intestines it takes with it the bile produced by the liver and the cholesterol contained in the food. The fiber or cellulose keeps the body from reabsorbing these potentially dangerous substances. So there is also an effect on the lowering of blood cholesterol. People who eat large amounts of carbohydrate and meat with little or no roughage show a higher incidence of colon cancer. The meat and starches tend to stagnate in the intestinal tract, since they do not stimulate intestinal motility to evacuate them. As a result, there are poisonous waste products from the putrefaction of these "hung-up" foods, which come in contact with the intestinal lining regularly and for prolonged periods.

What's wrong with meat? As soon as the animal is killed, the flesh begins to decay. As the animals are being killed, they all sense this and build up a tremendous fear which releases adrenalin into their tissues, which is eaten by the consumer. Most animals are given DES (diethylstilbestrol), a synthetic female sex hormone, to put on abnormal weight. The consumer eats the meat, including the hormone, and this has been known to cause serious problems, particularly in women. The end products of meat digestion and putrefaction in the intestinal tract are such poisons as skatol, indol, phenol, acetic acid, and uric acid, all of which tend to poison the body. The uric acid is responsible for gout and gouty arthritis as well as kidney stones.

Man is not carnivorous. If he was, there would be no problem with meat eating. However, many facts stand out to show he is non-carnivorous. A few of these are: The carnivore has an enzyme—uricase—which renders uric acid harmless. The carnivore has a short intestinal canal, while man's is extremely long allowing meat (which is highly putrefactive) to decay even further on its long trip to the outside world. The carnivore possesses claws; man has flat nails. The carnivore has a rasping tongue, man does not. The carnivore has pointed molar teeth for tearing, while man has blunt molar teeth for grinding. The carnivorous animal has no pores; he perspires through the mouth (panting). Man and the other non-carnivorous animals, with the exception of the elephant, have pores and perspire through the skin.

Also, as an animal lives and eats it must constantly give off waste products of metabolism or it will die of its own poisons. When the consumer eats the flesh, he is eating also the waste products of metabolism, which is a part of the meat and still in it. This predisposes to many of man's diseases.

Proper foods do not cure. They give to the body all the essential elements it needs to maintain its natural immunities, its health, and its optimum function. It is through the improper combining of foods—the haphazard habit of putting anything and everything into one's stomach—that is a cause of many of our ills, both minor and life-threatening. The purpose of food combining is to facilitate digestion—to make it easier, less complicated, and more efficient, even in the presence of some so-called digestive problems. We have certain physiological (functional) limitations of the digestive system (glands, enzymes, juices) and the digestion of different foods requires special adaptations in the digestive secretions.

Based on the principles of the chemistry of digestion, here are the rules of proper food combining:

1. Never eat carbohydrate (starch) and acid foods at the same meal. Don't eat bread, potatoes, rice, etc., with oranges, grapefruit, tomatoes, pineapple, etc. The salivary enzyme ptyalin, which begins starch digestion in the mouth, is alkaline in nature and is neutralized or destroyed by mild acids, even to the extent of 0.003 percent. If this occurs, then starch digestion is delayed and these foods begin to decompose in the stomach and produce gas and noxious chemicals.

2. Never eat a concentrated protein and a concentrated starch (carbohydrate) at the same meal. This means do not eat such items as nuts, meat, eggs, cheese, etc., with such items as bread, potatoes, rice, cereals, etc. Probably the most common example is meat and potatoes, or even a hamburger or hot dog sandwich. Next to overeating, this particularly bad combination is probably responsible for more digestive problems and eventual illness than any other abusive food combination. The digestion of starches and proteins is so different, that when they are indiscriminately mixed in the stomach, the digestion of each is interfered with. The protein digestion requires an acid

medium in the stomach while the starch digestion, which begins in the mouth, takes place in an alkaline medium. The starch digestion cannot be carried on for long because the increasing stomach acidity soon stops or slows up starch digestion and this results in putrefaction, gas, and toxic end products of this decomposition. As a result, the "average" person eating the "average" meal of many courses usually comes away from the table with the usual fullness, bloating, gas, and, later on, foul stools.

3. Never eat two different concentrated proteins at the same meal. For example, don't eat nuts and meat, eggs and meat, nuts and cheese, cheese and eggs, etc., at one meal. Two proteins of different types and compositions require different types of digestive juices of varying strength and character pouring into the stomach at different times, thus reducing the efficiency of digestion. Since people eat more than one or two meals and since there is protein in almost everything eaten in the properly balanced diet, one does not have to consume all of his proteins in any one meal. This doesn't mean that several types of meat or nuts or cheese cannot be eaten at one meal, except this usually leads to overeating.

4. Don't eat fats with proteins. This means do not mix cream, butter, oil, etc., with meat, eggs, cheese, nuts, etc. Fat hinders gastric (stomach) digestion. It lessens the amount of gastric juice secreted. It keeps the enzymes from attacking the food by encasing the food particles. Fat also lowers the amount of pepsin and hydrochloric acid in the gastric juice.

5. Do not eat acid foods and protein at the same meal. For example, oranges, tomatoes, lemons, pineapple, grapefruit, etc., should not be eaten with meat, cheese,

eggs, nuts, etc. These acids, instead of assisting in protein digestion as many people erroneously think, actually retard protein digestion and this results in putrefaction, since an unhampered flow of gastric juices is imperatively demanded by protein foods. Even vinegar used on salads serves as a check to hydrochloric acid secretion and this interferes with protein digestion, because hydrochloric acid activates pepsin. The two exceptions to this rule would be the use of cheese and nuts with the acid foods because these foods contain enough fat to inhibit gastric secretion for a longer time than do acids. Also, these two foods do not decompose as quickly as other protein foods when they are not immediately digested.

The simple fact is that the less complex our food mixtures and the simpler our meals, then the more efficient may we expect digestion to be. There have been so many people who have not changed their way of life or diet, but just observed the proper food combining rules and have noticed remarkable improvement in their digestion, in their health, and general well-being.

Actually it is not ideal to eat the easily digested foods such as the fruits with the more concentrated and heavy proteins, because the fruits are held up during digestion of protein in the stomach. This can tie up the fruit in the stomach for a number of hours, during which time the fruit decomposes and causes much gas and discomfort. It is better to eat the fruit first, wait maybe 15 minutes or so and then eat the concentrated, heavier protein food. In fact, as a general rule one should eat the less concentrated food such as fruit or vegetables first, and the concentrated foods of starches and protein last.

6. Ideally, melons and all the other countless fruits

and berries should be eaten at a fruit meal alone—nothing else, just the fruit. Many people say they can't eat melons or whatever fruit because they get gas and feel bloated. Well one of the greatest dietetic sins these people commit is the eating of these melons, etc., as a cool, refreshing dessert after a "hearty" meal. This fruit *has* to rot and decompose while it is held up in the stomach waiting for all of this other digestion to take place. Never eat fruit as a dessert.

7. Don't eat sugars and proteins at the same meal. These hinder protein digestion in the stomach because all sugars (commercial sugar, honey, sweet fruits such as dates, figs, etc.) have an inhibiting effect on the secretion of gastric juice and upon motility of the stomach. If sugars are eaten alone, they pass quickly into the intestine, but when eaten with other foods (proteins and starches), they are held up in the stomach for a prolonged period awaiting digestion of the other foods, and so they undergo decomposition.

8. Do not eat starches and sugars together at the same meal. This means breads, cereals, potatoes, rice, pastries, etc., with jams or jellies, syrup, sugared products, honey, etc. All sugars are readily dispatched from the stomach, but if eaten with other foods, such as the starches, they are held up in the stomach while awaiting the starch digestion and this causes decomposition of the sugar, with formation of gas and bloating. Most important is the fact that when sugars and starches are taken into the mouth, the mouth fills with saliva, but it doesn't contain the enzyme ptyalin because ptyalin does not act on sugars; or the saliva may contain very little ptyalin insuring that starch digestion will either not take place or will be in-

terfered with, causing gas, bloating, and toxic products. One of the worst abominations is pancakes and syrup.

I'm sure most of you know that full, bloated, and gassy feeling after eating a large meal that violates the principles of proper food combining. Very few people go away from the table feeling comfortable. In fact, most people get that tired, heavy, sluggish feeling that makes them drowsy after a "graciously" prepared meal.

9. Eat but one concentrated starch food at a meal. This is not because there is any conflict in the digestion of these foods, but because taking two or more concentrated starches at a meal is practically certain to lead to overeating of these foods, which usually leads to decomposition with its toxic end products.

The following classification of foods will make it easier to understand and use the principles of food combining that have been presented. The lists are by no means complete, but should be sufficient as a base from which to begin. From your reading, you know which foods to use and you know which foods not to use. You know which foods will build health and which foods will not; therefore, the list will not contain any "junk" foods. There will be a few foods not hygienic, but these will be used for clarification, although some may use them occasionally, particularly those who feel they cannot change their habits too quickly and must go through a transition period. Many foods contain both protein and carbohydrate.

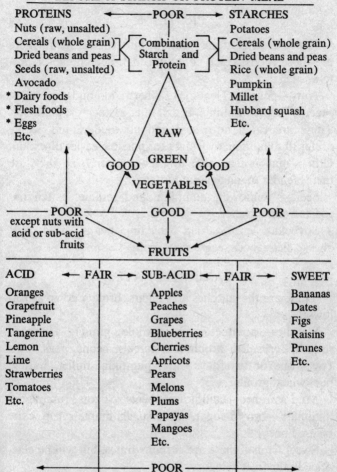

BASIC GUIDE TO CORRECT FOOD COMBINING †
MAY EAT STEAMED NON-STARCH VEGETABLES BEFORE A STARCH OR PROTEIN MEAL

PROTEINS ← POOR → STARCHES

Combination Starch and Protein

PROTEINS	STARCHES
Nuts (raw, unsalted)	Potatoes
Cereals (whole grain)	Cereals (whole grain)
Dried beans and peas	Dried beans and peas
Seeds (raw, unsalted)	Rice (whole grain)
Avocado	Pumpkin
* Dairy foods	Millet
* Flesh foods	Hubbard squash
* Eggs	Etc.
Etc.	

RAW GREEN VEGETABLES

GOOD — GOOD

POOR (except nuts with acid or sub-acid fruits) — GOOD — POOR

FRUITS

ACID ← FAIR → SUB-ACID ← FAIR → SWEET

ACID	SUB-ACID	SWEET
Oranges	Apples	Bananas
Grapefruit	Peaches	Dates
Pineapple	Grapes	Figs
Tangerine	Blueberries	Raisins
Lemon	Cherries	Prunes
Lime	Apricots	Etc.
Strawberries	Pears	
Tomatoes	Melons	
Etc.	Plums	
	Papayas	
	Mangoes	
	Etc.	

← POOR →

EAT FRUITS OR RAW VEGETABLES FIRST, FOLLOWED BY THE MORE CONCENTRATED FOODS (STARCH OR PROTEIN) LAST

†Adapted from the "Correct Food Combining Chart" by the Shangri-La Natural Hygiene Institute, Bonita Springs, Florida.

* Included for clarity but not recommended (although some may use cheese as a compromise food).

PROTEINS

Every food contains protein, but what is meant here are those foods which contain a high percentage of protein, such as:

Nuts—peanuts (legume), filberts, almonds, cashews, pecans, English walnuts, Brazil nuts, pistachios, pignolias, These are eaten unroasted and unsalted. Some people prefer to soak them overnight for possible easier digestion. Others may not be able to chew properly, so they use their blender to make a nut butter.

Seeds—sunflower, pumpkin, and sesame. Eaten unroasted and unsalted.

Soybeans, lentils, dried baby lima beans, dried peas, cheese, flesh foods, eggs, meat, milk.

CARBOHYDRATES

These are the starches and sugars, broken down as follows:

Starches—potatoes, rice (whole grain), Hubbard squash, Jerusalem artichokes, cereals, beans, peas, corn (over one or two days old), pumpkin, millet, barley, buckwheat groats.

Mild starches—cauliflower, beets, carrots, rutabaga.

Sugars—brown sugar, white sugar, maple syrup, cane syrup, honey.

Sweet fruits—these are carbohydrates, but will be classified in the fruit category.

FATS

Olive oil, soy oil, sunflower seed oil, sesame oil, nut oils (should be unprocessed and cold-pressed), butter, cream, butter substitutes, avocados. Many nuts contain fats.

ACID FRUITS (CITRUS)

Oranges, grapefruit, pineapple, lemons, limes, tomatoes, strawberries, tangerines.

SUB-ACID FRUITS

Peaches, apples, nectarines, pears, papaya, mango, apricots, fresh figs, sweet cherries and plums, blueberries, grapes.

SWEET FRUITS

Bananas, dried fruits such as figs, dates, raisins, and prunes. The dried fruits should be sun-dried, unsprayed, and unbleached. Persimmons may also be included here.

MELONS

These can be classified as sub-acid fruits: watermelon, honeydew, casaba, cantaloupe, crenshaw, muskmelon.

Do not eat acid and sweet fruits together as the sugar from the sweet fruits may ferment.

NON-STARCHY AND GREEN VEGETABLES

This group comprises the longest list regardless of the vegetable color classification, such as red, yellow, green, or white.

Lettuce (preferably leaf lettuce such as Romaine), broccoli, Brussels sprouts, collards, celery, cabbage, Chinese cabbage, eggplant, cucumber, green beans, spinach, okra, zucchini and yellow summer squash, leeks, onions, sweet pepper, chard, beet and turnip tops, asparagus, sprouts such as alfalfa, mung bean, lentil, etc., radish, rhubarb, parsley, kale, fresh-picked corn (which becomes a starch one day after it has been picked), endive, escarole, fresh peas.

The following are a few samples of properly combined protein meals:

Vegetable salad
Steamed asparagus
Yellow summer or zucchini squash
Nuts

Vegetable salad
Steamed broccoli
Green beans
Cottage or Ricotta cheese

Vegetable salad
Spinach
Fresh green peas
Sunflower seeds

Grapefruit
Nuts

Oranges
Unprocessed cheese

Grapefruit and orange
Nuts or seeds or cheese

Pineapple and orange
Avocado

The following are a few samples of properly combined starch meals:

Vegetable salad
Green beans
Kale
Potatoes

Vegetable salad
Zucchini squash
Asparagus
Brown rice

Vegetable salad
Spinach
Fresh peas
Yams

Vegetable salad
Broccoli
Beet greens
Millet or Hubbard squash

The following are a few samples of properly combined fruit meals:

Oranges	Dates	Orange	Peach
Grapefruit	Apples	Apple	Plum
	Pears	Grapes	Figs

Oranges
Pineapple

Apples	Peach	Berries	Peach
Grapes	Apple	Grapes	Grapes
Papaya	Banana	Pear	Dates

There are some times when a colitis (or other digestive disease) victim cannot or should not fast, but still needs adequate and life-giving nutrition. Although a basically raw vegetarian diet may not be able to be handled by the active, unhealed colitis case—because of the course roughage—I have found that the use of fresh-made vegetable juice followed by a blended salad two or three times a day *before* each meal has given marvelous results.

Since many colitis victims are physically depleted, this little regime allows and adds food that can more easily be handled and absorbed by the body, supplying it with proper and vital nutrients such as minerals, vitamins, carbohydrates, and chlorophyll protein so the body can be built up again. This juice and blended salad regime is relatively simple. You need a juicer (centrifugal type) and a blender.

The juices can be made as follows: 2 ounces tomato and 6 ounces celery juice (preferably twice daily); 2 ounces tomato and 6 ounces cucumber juice (once daily). Once every few days you can alternate the tomato-cucumber juice with 2 ounces carrot and 2 ounces celery juice.

The amount of blended salad should be about 8–12 ounces each time and should contain approximately ½–¾ of a cucumber, ½–¾ of a green pepper, 4–6 Romaine lettuce leaves, and 1 or 2 pieces of celery which can be used to push the vegetables into the blades and after which can be allowed to drop into the blender.

Romaine lettuce and celery are good additions to fruit meals without violating proper combining; or a larger green salad would be preferable for a more complete nutritional balance. The salad can be pureed in a blender for those with chewing difficulties.

The following are a number of sample menus and are intended as guides to help you understand the food combining principles and allow you to plan and create your own menus. It is important not to establish inflexible menus with little variety; anything by rote will become monotonous. You should learn to make meals from whatever is on hand. Believe it or not, you can create vegetarian culinary masterpieces after a while, just as we have done at home. It is not only a challenge, it is fun. It is important to keep the meals simple, but there are times you might want some fancy vegetarian dish such as eggplant parmigiana, steamed cauliflower au gratin, lentil loaf with vegetables, mashed potatoes and corn casserole, vegetable chop suey, corn or rice stuffed peppers, various steamed vegetable stews, stuffed cabbage with rice and vegetables, etc. You can take almost any standard recipe from any book and convert it to a vegetarian dish without violating the principles of food combining.

Remember, the most basic and important part of a meal is the fresh, raw natural foods. They take preference over cooked foods and should be the largest part of the meal, preventing you from overeating the cooked foods.

Once you have become familiar with food combining, the practice will become automatic and you will not have to spend much time on it. However, don't become a neurotic on the subject; don't split hairs. If you're out with friends, eat your meal, enjoy it, and forget it. Don't give lectures at the dining table. Everything can't be perfect, and if some combinations are not just right, you'll find that after you have finished the meal you will still be alive. Too many people are so busy analyzing their food and their bowel movements that life passes them by. Don't become one of them.

BREAKFASTS

Watermelon or other melon

One grapefruit
Two oranges
3 or 4 ounces of nuts or seeds

One grapefruit
One orange

One apple
Six dates
Two bananas

Whole canteloupe
Dish of berries

Three oranges
Cheese

Fresh carrot and celery juice
Or fresh tomato and celery juice

Two apples
Two peaches
Grapes
Raisins

Fresh pineapple
Two oranges
3 or 4 ounces of nuts or cheese

Ideally, and contrary to "popular opinion," it is better to omit breakfast. We don't need all the food we think we do and this limits overeating. However, if you desire breakfast then by all means eat it. Children are growing, so they should have breakfast. But after your body adjusts itself to this type of diet (and there is an adjustment, be it some initial weight loss or whatever), try omitting breakfast once in a while. You may be pleasantly surprised at how much better you will feel.

LUNCHES

These can be fruit-type meals as covered under breakfasts or vegetable-type meals as will be listed. I feel that the majority of lunches should be the vegetable-type with emphasis on the ever-important salads with lots of Romaine lettuce and other life-giving greens.

When the term "salad" is used, it is understood to include (depending on whether a protein or a starch meal is to be eaten) a large and abundant variety of raw, fresh vegetables, such as: plenty of Romaine and/or leaf lettuce, celery, cucumber, carrots, sweet pepper, cabbage, tomatoes, fresh sprouts, avocado, cauliflower, fresh peas, and whatever else you might want to toss into it. The salad should be eaten whole and uncut, but if you prefer a tossed salad, then alternate between the two. When you chop the vegetables, they are more quickly oxidized and lose some of their nutritive values.

Vegetable salad
Orange
Apple
3 or 4 ounces of nuts,
    or unprocessed cheese,
    or one avocado

Vegetable salad
String beans
Brown rice with vegetables

Three tomatoes
4 or 5 ounces of Ricotta
    cheese or washed cottage cheese

Vegetable salad
Steamed asparagus
Steamed kale
Two sweet potatoes

Vegetable salad
Steamed broccoli
Turnip greens
Hubbard squash

Vegetable salad
Two ears of corn

Peas
Two steamed or baked potatoes

Very large tossed
    vegetable salad with 3 or 4
    ounces of cheese chopped
    into it

Vegetable salad
One avocado

Vegetable salad
Steamed yellow squash
3 or 4 ounces of nuts or seeds

SUPPER

This can be similar to the lunches with emphasis on the raw salads; however, you may switch the meals around if you prefer—e.g., the breakfasts can become suppers if you prefer fruit at that time. The important fact is that you eat a well-rounded and balanced variety of all the food types during the course of a day.

Vegetable salad
Steamed acorn squash
Lentil stew

Vegetable salad
Steamed zucchini squash
Eggplant Parmigiana

Vegetable salad
Spinach
Okra
Soy bean loaf

Vegetable salad
Steamed peas
Two steamed or baked potatoes

Vegetable salad
Steamed green beans
3 or 4 ounces of nuts

Vegetable salad
Steamed eggplant, tomato and okra
4 or 5 ounces of cheese (Ricotta or a raw milk, salt-free
cheese)

If you don't wish to give up flesh foods just yet, then substitute meat or fish occasionally where the meal calls for protein, but don't eat any flesh foods with fruit or starches.

Again, for a well-rounded nutritional impact, you may use a fresh green (non-starch) salad to be eaten before any meal containing fruit. If there's a chewing problem, put the salad in a blender and puree it. In fact, for anyone with a chewing problem, use the blended salad at any meal.

The varieties of foods are unlimited and you should have no problem enjoying your creations; and if you can, take that 36-hour fast once a week.

I've tried to give you some basic principles, some tools

with which to rebuild your life, enjoy vigorous health, and probably even add a few years to a life which is all too short. You must read and you must analyze, but most important and perhaps the most difficult thing for you to do first is to change your way of thinking—flexibility and open-mindedness.

There were many men in past history who were so far ahead of their time as to be ridiculed by their peers and others. I should like to quote from some of these famous people:

William Shakespeare—"They are as sick that surfeit with too much, as they that starve with nothing."

Thomas Edison—"Natural foods will be the medicine of the future."

Oliver Wendell Holmes, M.D. (poet, novelist, physician)—In his address to the Massachusetts Medical Society, May 30, 1860: "I firmly believe that if all the (drugs and medicines) as now used could be sunk to the bottom of the sea, it would be all the better for mankind and all the worse for the fishes."

Benjamin Franklin—"He is the best physician that knows the worthlessness of most medicines." Also, "A full belly is the mother of all evil." Finally, "Many dishes, many diseases. Many medicines, few cures."

Dr. Keki Sidhwa, one of our Natural Hygiene professionals from England, was quoted in the June, 1971, Hygienic Review: "Natural Hygiene is not something you are following by rule of thumb. It is an experience in living; a dynamic rather than a static, dry list of invariable rules. The needs of the body can vary from day to day and to live Hygienically you have to meet these variations when they occur. If you do not do so, your body will fall asleep and you may exist but you will not thrive."

So what then is the philosophy of Natural Hygiene?

Natural Hygiene revolves around one word—"life." All life is precious; all life is a learning experience. Life is our teacher and we are its pupils. For it is only in life, not death, that lessons can be learned. Life can also be a severe taskmaster so that we may each evolve toward that truth and perfection that we ultimately seek. Natural Hygiene is a way of life, not a collection of assorted cures. There are no "cures." It is a beautiful mode of living. It is a system of care of the mind and body in sickness and in health, based upon recognition and dedication to unerring laws of nature. It demonstrates the principle that all good, all enduring happiness and all true progress are found only in obedience to these laws of life. Natural Hygiene is a way of life that allows those who have health to maintain it; it allows those who have lost health to regain it; and it allows those who have never had health to experience it.

Modern Natural Hygiene is a revival. In its essential elements, it was practiced by primeval man as a way of life. It belonged to him as it belongs to the lower animals. The animals retain those built-in instincts, selecting what is good for them and rejecting what is not. Man, however, has lost his natural instinct after years of artificial ways of living and eating and after years of "overcivilization." Today, Natural Hygiene is based upon the sciences of physiology and biology.

The laws of life and nature are unchanging. It is man who must change. The laws of life are perfect, but man is imperfect and must acquire knowledge and awareness so that he may apply these perfect laws of life and find health and contentment. Man cannot duplicate nature. Man must work in harmony with natural laws.

A true science of life, which Natural Hygiene seeks to establish, can arise only out of a study of life and man and not out of a study of chemistry. A true science of life will not come out of the laboratory alone, but must be based primarily upon a study of man as a living, feeling, thinking, acting being. It is the responsibility—indeed it is the mission—of all people to discover and understand the laws of life and to understand the results of violating these immutable laws. Wrong living is the beginning of disease and weakness. Right living is the foundation of health and strength. Health and disease are not gifts of nature. They are not the results of chance. These are conditions you choose and build for yourself.

Hygiene is a total awareness encompassing every facet of our lives, and it begins every day and with every precious breathing moment that we live. We must make ourselves consciously aware and give our attention to all of the basic principles that have been presented in this book (and to those additional principles you will learn in your further reading).

Our occupations, habits and environment all affect our lives. We must be constantly aware of our emotions and make efforts to discipline our anger and negative inclinations. We must be aware of every word we say and every thought we think. We must be positive in thought, kind, sympathetic, loving, and unselfish. Hygiene helps us become aware. Hygiene gives our bodies the healthy environment we need to make ourselves better and better every day and in every way. And that is why we are here, is it not? We are altogether seeking knowledge. Because of our limitations, we are seeking to perfect ourselves— and that is good. To seek self-understanding, self-improvement, and self-perfection is the highest achievement of man. We should treat our body like a holy temple. We should revere it with awe and respect and never do or say anything to degrade it, to harm it, or poison it. It is true we must love ourselves first before we can love others, but to love ourselves first, we must, as Socrates said, "Know thyself."

In the final analysis, it all depends upon you and the degree to which you can apply these principles and make them work for you. All the knowledge in the world is useless unless you put it into daily, living practice. Try not to limit yourselves, for Natural Hygiene is not a life of denial, but rather it is a life of fulfillment.

If this book has aroused your curiosity, stimulated your interest, or motivated you in any way, then its only purpose has been realized.

Recommended Reading

Information about the American Natural Hygiene Society and the following books can be obtained from the: American Natural Hygiene Society, 1920 Irving Park Road, Chicago, Illinois   60613.

Fasting Can Save Your Life
Health for the Millions
The Greatest Health Discovery
Dictionary of Man's Foods
Exercise
Hygienic Care of Children
Natural Hygiene: Man's Pristine Way of Life
You Don't Have to Be Sick
Introduction to Natural Hygiene
The Hygienic System, Volume II (Food and Feeding)
The Hygienic System, Volume III (Fasting)
Human Beauty: Its Culture and Hygiene
Food Combining Made Easy
Rubies in the Sand
Superior Nutrition
Living Life to Live It Longer
Fasting for Health and Long Life

Toxemia—The Basic Cause of All Disease
Fit Food for Man
Fasting for Renewal of Life
Medical Drugs on Trial
Homemakers' Guide to Foods for Pleasure and Health

Bibliography

Aring, Charles D. "Primum Non Nocere," *Archives of Internal Medicine*, Volume 115, March, 1965, pp. 345–350.

Bagdade, John D., and Porte, Daniel Jr., and Bierman, Edwin L. "Steroid-Induced Lipemia," *Archives of Internal Medicine*, Volume 125, January, 1970, pp. 129–134.

Bakulev, A.N., and Kolesnikova, R.S. "Starvation Treatment (Preliminary Report)," *Klinicheskaia Meditsina*, Volume 40, Number 2, February, 1962, pp. 14–21.

Ball, Michael F., and Canary, John J., and Kyle, Laurence H. "Tissue Changes During Intermittent Starvation and Caloric Restriction as Treatment for Severe Obesity," *Archives of Internal Medicine*, Volume 125, January, 1970, pp. 62–68.

Best, Charles Herbert, and Taylor, Norman Burke. *Physiological Basis of Medical Practice*, 8th edition, Williams and Wilkins Co., Baltimore, 1966, pp. 550, 1405-1407.

"Breaking The Obesity Barrier," *Medical World News*, Volume 3, Number 15, July 20, 1962, pp. 75–76.

Cahill, George F., and Aoki, Thomas T. "How Metabolism Affects Clinical Problems," *Resident and Staff Physician*, April, 1973, p. 32.

Crile, George. *Cancer and Common Sense*, Viking Press, New York, 1955, p. 42.

"Dramatic Treatment For Obesity; Diseased Patients Test

Starvation Diet," *Journal of the American Medical Association*, Volume 197, Number 1, July 4, 1966, p. 22.

Duncan, Garfield G., et al. "Correction and Control of Intractable Obesity," *Journal of the American Medical Association*, Volume 181, Number 4, July 28, 1962, pp. 309–312.

Fuchs, Victor R. "Can the Tradition and Practice of Medicine Survive?" *Archives of Internal Medicine*, Volume 125, January, 1970, pp. 154–156.

Hawk, Philip Bovier, and Oser, Bernard L., and Summerson, William H. *Practical Physiological Chemistry*, 12th edition, Blakiston Co., Philadelphia, 1947, p. 971.

Hunter, Beatrice Trum. *Consumer Beware*, Bantam Books, New York, 1972.

————. *Food Additives and Your Health*, Keats Publishing Co., New Canaan, Connecticut, 1972.

Jagasia, K.H., and Thurman, William G. "Wilm's Tumor in the Adult," *Archives of Internal Medicine*, Volume 115, March, 1965, pp. 322–325.

Longgood, William. *The Poisons in Your Food*, Pyramid Books, New York, 1969.

Moore, Frederick J. "Information Technologies and Health Care," *Archives of Internal Medicine*, Volume 125, January, 1970, pp. 157–161.

"Obesity," *World-Wide Abstracts of General Medicine*, Volume 9, Number 5, June, 1966, p. 22.

Plant Foods for Human Nutrition, Pergamon Press, New York and England, Volume 1, Numbers 1,2,3,4, May 1968, February 1969, June 1969, November 1969, and Volume 2, Numbers 1,2,3,4, June 1970, January 1971, March 1972 (numbers 3 & 4).

Rosenberg, Benjamin A., and Bloom, Walter, and Spencer, Herta. "Three Views of the Treatment and Hazards of Obesity," *Journal of the American Medical Associa-*

tion, Volume 186, Number 7, November 16, 1963, pp. 43–53.

Shelton, Herbert M. *Fasting Can Save Your Life*, Natural Hygiene Press, Chicago, 1973.

———. *Food Combining Made Easy*, Dr. Shelton's Health School, San Antonio, 1975.

———. *The Hygienic System, Volume 2*, Dr. Shelton's Health School, San Antonio, 1969.

———. *The Hygienic System, Volume 3*, Dr. Shelton's Health School, San Antonio, 1969.

———. *Superior Nutrition*, Dr. Shelton's Health School, San Antonio, 1970.

"Starving Therapy for Refractory Obesity," *Modern Medicine*, May 3, 1971, p. 77.

White, Abraham, and Handler, Philip, and Smith, Emil L. *Principles of Biochemistry*, 4th edition, McGraw-Hill, New York, 1968, p. 628.

Young, Vernon R., and Scrimshaw, Nevin S. "The Physiology of Starvation," *Scientific American*, Volume 225, Number 4, October, 1971, pp. 14–21.

Zoethout, William D., and Tuttle, W.W. *Textbook of Physiology*, 9th edition, C.V. Mosby Co., St. Louis, 1948.

Index